Praise for
Could It Be B12?

"In this long-needed book, Pacholok and Stuart expose a major health-care scandal: the failure to identify and treat hundreds of thousands of patients who suffer from vitamin B_{12} deficiency. The cost: an epidemic of dementia, heart disease, depression, developmental disability, infertility, and neurological disorders that doctors write off as "diabetic neuropathy," "multiple sclerosis-like symptoms," or "just old age."

In exposing this scandal and explaining how simply we can stop it, the authors provide an invaluable service for medical consumers who want to protect their families and for all medical care providers who truly care about their patients. An important, highly recommended contribution."

—Bernard Rimland, Ph.D.
　　Director, Autism Research Institute

"Its been said that nothing is so blind as the eye that wills not to see. As a practicing physician I can only hope that malpractice attorneys don't read this book."

—Richard Nimbach, D.O.

"I defy you to read this book, then *not* get yourself or a loved one tested for B12 deficiency."

—Dr. Eric Norman, developer of the uMMA test for B_{12} deficiency and founder of the first commercial laboratory to provide uMMA testing

"Vitamin B_{12} deficiency is an epidemic causing more health damage than the polio epidemic and it can now be prevented through screening and treatment."

—Sally M. Pacholok, R.N.

Could ItBe B12 ?

An Epidemic of Misdiagnoses

by
Sally M. Pacholok, R.N.
Jeffrey J. Stuart, D.O.

*Published by Quill Driver Books
an imprint of Linden Publishing
2006 S. Mary
Fresno, California 93721
559-233-6633 • 1-800-345-4447 • FAX 559-233-6933
QuillDriverBooks.com
Info@QuillDriverBooks.com*

Quill Driver Books' titles may be purchased in quantity at special
discounts for educational, fund-raising, business, or promotional use. Please
contact Special Markets, Quill Driver Books/Word Dancer Press, Inc. at the
above address or at **1-800-345-4447**.

Project Cadre:
Doris Hall, Dave Marion, Mary McBroom, Stephen Blake Mettee

ISBN: 1-884956-46-7 • 978-1884956-46-1

57986

Printed in the United States of America

QUILL DRIVER BOOKS and COLOPHON ARE TRADEMARKS OF LINDEN PUBLISHING, INC.

To order another copy of this book, please call
1-800-345-4447.

Library of Congress Cataloging-in Publication Data

Pacholok, Sally M., 1963-
Could it be b12?: an epidemic of misdiagnoses / by Sally M. Pacholok, Jeffrey J. Stuart.
p. cm.
ISBN 1-884956-46-7 (trade pbk.)
1. Vitamin B12 deficiency--Popular works. I. Stuart, Jeffrey J., 1965- II. Title.
RC627.V55P33 2005
614.5'9396--dc22

2005006106

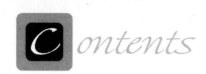

This book is dedicated to all those who are presently suffering, have suffered, are injured, disabled, institutionalized, or have died because of the continued misdiagnosis of vitamin B_{12} deficiency.

For my father
Andrew William Pacholok
and
In memory of my mother
Anna June Nykiforuk-Pacholok

For my favorite "B_{12} Buddies"
Susan Stuart, Mary Stuart, Milton Lute, Jean Lute, Peggy Demmin,
Johnny Leone, Jim Mundy, Norbert Biebuyck, Dale Back,
Charlene Back, and Barb Darga

Sometimes it takes an individual afflicted with a disease to make positive changes, create awareness, and become an advocate for others who are suffering.

Please note: The names of patients mentioned in this book have been changed to respect patient confidentiality.

Acknowledgments

We would especially like to thank the many dedicated scientists, researchers, and clinicians who have contributed a vast amount of medical literature over the last century regarding vitamin B_{12} deficiency.

We are very grateful to our editor, Stephen Blake Mettee at Quill Driver Books, who recognized the importance of making the public aware of this crucial health issue and enabled us to make this book a reality. Special thanks also to Alison Blake for her hard work and good humor in the face of innumerable changes and additions of new research.

Our personal thanks to Joseph Flynn, D.O. and Richard Nimbach, D.O., who took the time to read our manuscript, understand the epidemic of undiagnosed B_{12} deficiency, and actually test patients in their current practice in order to improve patient care. I am indebted as well to Dr. Bernard Rimland, for his invaluable support and encouragement. Private thanks to Anna Pijanowska, Sue Harvey, Alice Vandemergle, and Karen Balaska-O'Donnell.

Introduction

In 1983, I was the picture of health. I looked fit, I felt great, and I had no idea that a silent crippler lurked inside me, stealthily damaging my brain, nerves, blood vessels, and in fact nearly every organ in my body.

Because of my medical training, however, I noticed small signs that something wasn't right, and I knew enough to be worried even when my doctors dismissed those signs as "nothing to worry about." I pursued the few clues that my potentially deadly disease left, eventually obtaining a diagnosis of pernicious anemia (an autoimmune form of vitamin B_{12} deficiency), and as a result I'll never suffer the terrible symptoms that this disorder can cause.

Millions of other victims of B_{12} deficiency—many of them also victims of doctors who mistakenly ruled out B_{12} deficiency with serum B_{12} tests or blood smears, or never considered the diagnosis at all—aren't as lucky. Some are infants and toddlers, left developmentally disabled for life. Some are young adults, mistakenly diagnosed as having multiple sclerosis or told, erroneously, that they are "incurably" infertile. Others are middle-aged men and women, tormented by balance problems, numb hands or feet, or mysterious shooting leg pains so agonizing that they can barely walk. Some are diagnosed with early-onset dementia or pre-Parkinson's disease in their thirties or forties. Some are people so depressed that they try to kill themselves. Some appear to be full-blown schizophrenics. And still others are seniors living out their days in nursing homes, because their doctors think they have Alzheimer's disease.

It's too late to completely reverse the symptoms of many of these people—but it's not too late to protect yourself, or the people you love, against a similarly tragic fate. In fact, it's extraordinarily simple to prevent or completely reverse the symptoms of B_{12} deficiency if the deficiency is discovered in time. But this condition isn't like other vitamin deficiencies, and simply taking a standard multivitamin pill won't always protect you; instead, you need an accurate diagnosis and medical treatment. And getting a diagnosis isn't always easy, as I know from experience.

I had no idea that an invisible disease was attacking my body when I went for a pre-employment physical examination back in 1983, when I was just nineteen. The first clue came when the examining physician reviewed my blood tests and commented on my abnormally large red blood cells. (In retrospect, I may owe my life to the fact that this test came back positive. Many people suffer neurological damage decades before their blood tests become abnormal, and by then it's too late.)

"What kind of diet do you eat?" the doctor asked when he saw my results. When I said that I didn't like vegetables, he told me to eat more of them, dismissing my blood abnormality as merely a sign of a diet low in folic acid.

One month later, another doctor commented again on my large red blood cells, but concluded that my lab results were "insignificant." Like the first doctor, this physician sent me on my way, unaware that he'd just missed diagnosing a disease that could destroy my brain, cripple my body, or even kill me.

Two years later, in nursing school, I bought a manual describing laboratory tests and their meanings. In the section on "macrocytosis"— the medical term for unusually large red blood cells—the manual outlined two different problems, folic acid deficiency and B$_{12}$ deficiency, which could cause this abnormality. Since I loved B$_{12}$-rich meat and didn't like folate-rich vegetables, I could see why my first doctor picked low folic acid as a likely culprit in my case. But I wondered why he'd never considered B$_{12}$ deficiency as well.

Thinking to myself, "It can't hurt to be sure," I persuaded a doctor at my hospital to order a serum folate and serum B$_{12}$ level for me. That night, when I mentioned the tests to my parents, my father surprised me by saying that my grandfather had been diagnosed with pernicious anemia—the most well-known, although *not* the most common, cause of B$_{12}$ deficiency—back in the 1960s. So I wasn't completely caught off-guard a few days later when my own B$_{12}$ test came back low. I started receiving B$_{12}$ shots, grateful that I'd obtained a diagnosis before I suffered any symptoms.

But that wasn't the end of my story. Two years later, when I needed surgery, I mentioned my B_{12} deficiency to my surgeon. Skeptical because she thought I was "awfully young" to have this problem, she sent me to a hematologist, who dismissed the idea that I had a B_{12} problem, in spite of my earlier diagnosis and positive findings. (In fact, the hematologist's chart notes, which I read surreptitiously at a later visit—a nurse's instinct!—suggested that I was merely a hysterical female, imagining problems that didn't exist.) I insisted he run tests anyway.

The hematologist had changed his mind by the time his office called me, a week later, asking me to come in "right away." By then, the tests he'd ordered had revealed that I indeed had juvenile pernicious anemia. In fact, he exclaimed exuberantly, I was the youngest patient he'd ever seen with pernicious anemia in his twenty years of practice. I felt like a rare freak of nature. This time around, the doctor was friendly and informative—and, I sensed, secretly relieved that I'd insisted he verify my earlier diagnosis. He certainly wouldn't have detected my problem on his own, even with all of the information I'd given him on my first visit, because that surreptitous glance at my chart showed that his suspected diagnoses *didn't even include* B_{12} deficiency.

In short, although I'd virtually handed this doctor my diagnosis, he nearly missed it. If I'd come to him without the benefit of my nursing training or without already knowing that I had a history of B_{12} deficiency, his failure could have injured or killed me—because, if I had passively accepted his initial opinion, I would have stopped receiving the B_{12} shots that saved my body from the ravages of pernicious anemia. And yet, in a way, I'm thankful to him.

Why? Because his disbelief led me to ponder an important question: How many other people suffer or die, because their doctors don't consider the simple diagnosis of B_{12} deficiency? I was lucky, because I had enlarged red blood cells—the easiest-to-spot sign of the problem—and a family history of pernicious anemia. Yet despite these red flags, this doctor, as well as others, missed the correct diagnosis. Unlike me, a third of people with B_{12} deficiency never develop either large red blood cells *or* anemia, meaning that their disease is invisible to routine blood tests. In addition, most have no known family history of B_{12} deficiency. I wondered: Were doctors misdiagnosing such patients on a regular basis?

My curiosity developed, over time, into nearly two decades of research on the scope of B_{12} deficiency. I became an expert, reading every textbook and journal article I could get my hands on, and making connections with both clinical doctors specializing in B_{12} deficiency and scientists involved in B_{12} research. My husband Jeffrey, an emergency medicine physician, also conducted research to determine the percentage of B_{12}-deficient patients seen in his emergency department. What we learned about the prevalence of B_{12} deficiency, the havoc it wreaks on the entire body, and the number of undiagnosed cases, is alarming.

B_{12} deficiency is very common—not just in seniors and middle-aged people, but even in teens, children, and infants. As many as 20 percent of people over sixty (and, according to one new study, 40 percent of seniors with severe mental or physical problems) are suffering, most of them unknowingly, from its ravages. Thousands of young children, teens, and young adults have borderline B_{12} levels, below what's considered necessary to keep their brains functioning optimally. And millions of people labeled as having Alzheimer's, multiple sclerosis, early-stage Parkinson's disease, autism, learning disability, depression, bipolar disorder, vision loss, schizophrenia, diabetic neuropathy, and other severe and often incurable disorders could actually be victims of the easily diagnosable, treatable, and (in its early stages) completely curable problem of B_{12} deficiency.

Initially I was tremendously excited by the extensive research proving that B_{12} deficiency plays a role in so many seemingly hopeless problems. That's because this is a problem that's simple to fix. It's an inexpensive problem as well, with treatment costing only a few dollars a month—pocket change, compared to the expense of other medical conditions. Thus, diagnosing and treating patients with B_{12} deficiency could both reduce the pain and suffering of these patients and cut medical care costs—a win-win situation, in my opinion.

My excitement was short-lived, however, because most of the doctors I worked with didn't care about an epidemic of undiagnosed B_{12} deficiency. They didn't care that the serum-B_{12} test available to diagnose the problem frequently was inaccurate and misleading. They didn't care about the growing number of journal articles warning about the high costs, both to patients and to society, of doctors' rampant failure to identify this problem. Indeed, they accused me of "playing doctor," and balked at ordering accurate B_{12} tests, even for patients with clear signs and symptoms of the disorder. Eventually, I was told, in no uncertain terms, to drop the subject or lose my job.

Their attitude didn't stem simply from the fact that I am a nurse, rather than a physician (although that didn't help). My husband encountered a similar level of apathy, even when he showed his colleagues study data revealing that large numbers of his own facility's patients suffered from undetected B_{12} deficiency. Later I learned that other physicians had encountered the same negative response from their own colleagues.

Faced with an impenetrable wall of apathy and eventually outright hostility, I slowly and quietly gave up. What else could I do? Those with the ability to diagnose and fight this disease chose instead to ignore it. Noted physicians had fought the battle to bring the B_{12}-deficiency epidemic to light, and had lost. What chance did I have of making a difference?

My silent surrender lasted until the day I was asked to discharge a patient who'd been labeled by the preceding shift as a "frequent flyer," a "drug-seeker," and a patient who "did not want to go home." When I examined this woman and reviewed her laboratory results and medical history, I saw painfully obvious indications of B_{12} deficiency—evidence that even a first-year medical student should be able to recognize. I also noted the complete absence of any effort by her doctors to test her accurately for this problem during her previous hospital admissions, or even to recommend such testing to her family physician. This sad and frightened woman had suffered for years from crippling and seemingly mysterious symptoms, *every one of which* could be explained by B_{12} deficiency, and yet no one had correctly evaluated her for the disorder. Instead, they'd simply labeled her as nuts.

She wasn't the first patient I'd seen dismissed by doctors who overlooked the signs and symptoms of B_{12} deficiency. In fact, she was only the latest in a long line of patients written off as hopeless by medical professionals who'd failed to diagnose a life-threatening, and very common, medical problem. Indeed, I'd seen far worse cases, including patients who were on the verge of death, or in a permanent state of dementia, as a result of undiagnosed B_{12} deficiency. Each case broke my heart. But this time, as I wrote up the discharge papers for this woman who'd received no real help and no real treatment—only a condescending response from her doctors and nurses, a large hospital bill, and a possible death sentence—my anger hit critical mass.

I knew that my own health and life had hung in the balance years earlier, when doctors told me that my troubling lab test findings were "insignificant." Now, on a regular basis, I was watching other patients being sentenced to death or disability by the doctors they trusted. I knew that many of these patients would wind up back in our hospital some day with strokes, dementia, depression, fall-caused fractures, the need for blood transfusions, and other problems stemming from undiagnosed B_{12} deficiency.

I could no longer stand by and be a silent accomplice to an epidemic of apathy and non-diagnosis that is leaving millions of young and old patients crippled or dead. As a medical professional, I'd long since come to terms with the daily tragedy of lives ruined by diseases that can't be prevented or cured. But I could not come to terms with the continuing parade of lives ruined by the failure to detect and treat a simple-to-identify, simple-to-treat, simple-to-cure disorder. Neither could my husband, a physician who finds it reprehensible to refuse a patient the couple of tests that could prevent nearly *every case* of disability or death due to B_{12} deficiency.

This book was born out of our frustration and anger over these lost lives. But it was also born out of hope—the hope that we can help many current and potential victims of B_{12} deficiency by putting this information in the hands of sufferers and their families, as well as in the hands of concerned medical professionals.

If you are a medical consumer, this book will empower you to protect yourself and your family members, by helping you to identify loved ones at risk for B_{12} deficiency, and to obtain a real diagnosis and real treatment before it's too late. And if you are a medical professional, we hope you will examine the compelling body of research reviewed in this book and make complete B_{12} screening (*not* just often-inaccurate serum B_{12} levels and blood smears) part of your standard practice. The hundreds of studies we cite, published in major and respected medical journals, prove that few diseases are more prevalent, simple to diagnose, and easy to treat than B_{12} deficiency—and few carry such a high, yet entirely preventable, risk of deadly disease or infirmity.

Above all, the message of this book is that the suffering caused by B_{12} deficiency, an "invisible" problem so pervasive that it touches the lives of nearly every family in America, is *unnecessary*. We can stop this cruel disorder in its tracks, before it destroys more lives. I dodged the bullet of B_{12} deficiency, and so can its other potential victims—but only if patients and doctors alike open their eyes to the scope of this hidden epidemic.

An Invisible Epidemic

A silent crippler stalks millions of Americans—and you may be one of them.

This crippler is a master of masquerade, striking different people in different ways. It afflicts one person with tremors, makes another depressed or psychotic, and causes agonizing leg and arm pains or paralysis in still another. It can mimic Alzheimer's disease, multiple sclerosis, early Parkinson's disease, diabetic neuropathy, or chronic fatigue syndrome. It can make men or women infertile, or cause developmental disabilities in their children. Other times, it lurks silently, stealthily increasing its victims' risk of deadly diseases, ranging from strokes and heart attacks to cancer.

This medical disorder stems from a vitamin deficiency, but your standard multivitamin pill won't prevent it in many cases, and even high-dose oral formulas of this vitamin may not help. It's considered an "old people's disease" by doctors, but it can strike any person at any age, and it sometimes hits children the hardest.

The disorder I've described is vitamin B_{12} deficiency. If you develop this deficiency, it's easy to spot, easy to treat, and easy to cure—but only if your doctor diagnoses you before it's too late. Unfortunately, that frequently doesn't happen.

Who are the victims of B_{12} deficiency?

The cases we'll describe in the pages of this book involve people of every age and from every walk of life: babies, young men and women, middle-aged people, and senior citizens.

Among them are the following:

- A thirty-five-year-old man who starts wetting himself, and who can no longer walk steadily or grip with his hands.

- An eight-month-old baby who loses her speech, stops responding to her parents, and eventually can't even sit up by herself.

- A twenty-year-old woman who becomes severely depressed, and who attempts to kill herself.

- A grandfather transformed, in three months, from a healthy jogger into a depressed, confused man, diagnosed with senile dementia.

- A young woman unable to conceive a baby.

- A fifty-four-year-old woman experiencing paranoid delusions and violent outbursts, coupled with symptoms that her doctor diagnoses as multiple sclerosis.

- An eighty-year-old man who develops balance problems, falls, and fractures his hip.

- A ballet dancer who undergoes cosmetic surgery and ends up nearly unable to walk.

- A middle-aged woman accused by her doctors of being an alcoholic and a "drug seeker" when she complains of intense, chronic back and leg pain.

- A seventy-eight-year-old with foot and leg numbness diagnosed as incurable diabetic neuropathy.

- A senior citizen whose doctors attribute his repeated falls to "mini-strokes."

All of these very different patients have one thing in common: Their doctors have failed to properly diagnose them. They've been labeled with a dozen different disorders, ranging from incurable diseases to hypochondria, but in reality, they all suffer from the same medical condition: vitamin B$_{12}$ deficiency.

This isn't a new or fad disease. In fact, you'll find it listed in the textbooks of any first-year medical student. It's not a rare disease, either: If you're over forty, you're at an elevated risk for dangerous B$_{12}$ deficiency, and if you're over sixty, you have up to a 40 percent chance of having potentially dangerous low B_{12} levels.

How Commom Is B_{12} Deficiency?

It's important to note that most of the studies mentioned below *underestimate* the prevalence of deficiency, because—as we'll explain later—many deficient people have normal serum B_{12} levels.

Tufts University researchers, analyzing data from the large-scale Framingham Offspring Study, found that *nearly 40 percent of participants between the ages of twenty-six and eighty-three* had plasma B_{12} levels in the "low normal" range—a level at which some people begin experiencing neurological symptoms. Nearly 9 percent had outright deficiency, and 16 percent exhibited near-deficiency. Remarkably, low serum B_{12} was as common in younger participants as in the elderly.[1]

Smaller studies report that 15 to 20 percent of seniors have a vitamin B_{12} deficiency.

A recent study found that 40 percent of hospitalized elderly patients had low or borderline serum B_{12} levels.[2]

Over 80 percent of long-term vegans who do not adequately supplement their diets with B_{12}, and over 50 percent of long-term vegetarians show evidence suggestive of B_{12} deficiency (see Chapter 6). [3, 4]

What is B_{12} and why is it so important?

To understand why B_{12} deficiency can hurt or even kill you, and why this deficiency is so common even in seemingly healthy people, it's important to know a little about what vitamins are—and why B_{12} is unique.

Your body needs thirteen different vitamins in order to stay alive and healthy. These tiny molecules participate in thousands of chemical reactions that build your tissues and organs, provide you with energy from the food you eat, clean the toxins from your body, protect you against infections, repair damage, and allow your cells to communicate with each other.

Your body can't make vitamins by itself, so it depends on you to provide them by eating the right foods. Some (the fat-soluble vitamins) can be stored; others, including the B vitamins, are water-soluble and need to be "restocked" every day. If you don't take in enough of a particular vitamin, your supplies dwindle, causing a marginal deficiency and, eventually, a deficiency disease such as scurvy (vitamin C deficiency) or beriberi (vitamin B$_1$ deficiency). The bigger the drain on your stores, the more serious the consequences will be—up to and including death.

Of the thirteen vitamins your body needs, one is vitamin B$_{12}$. It acts, in many ways, much like the other dozen vitamins. But in other important ways, vitamin B$_{12}$ is an oddity, and some of the quirks that make it different also make it harder for millions of people to get enough of it.

Among its distinctions, B$_{12}$ is the only vitamin that contains a trace element—cobalt—which explains its scientific name, *cobalamin*. Because B$_{12}$ is produced in the gut of animals, it's also the only vitamin that you can't obtain from plants or sunlight. Plants don't need B$_{12}$, so they don't produce or store it.* To obtain B$_{12}$ from your diet, you need to eat meat, poultry, fish, eggs, dairy products, or foods fortified with B$_{12}$—or, if you don't eat these foods, you need to take supplements. However, even a diet high in B$_{12}$, augmented with a supplement, isn't sufficient for many people.

In fact, while you need only a tiny, tiny amount of B$_{12}$ each day (two to four micrograms or about a millionth of an ounce), it's remarkably easy to become deficient in this nutrient. While deficiency often occurs in vegans or vegetarians who fail to take the right supplements, *the majority of B$_{12}$-deficient people eat plentiful amounts of the vitamin*—it's just that their bodies can't absorb or use it.

Why? Because to get from your mouth into your bloodstream, vitamin B$_{12}$ must follow a complex pathway, and a roadblock in any part of that pathway can cause your B$_{12}$ levels to plummet. Here's a highly simplified explanation of this pathway:

1. The vitamin B$_{12}$ in your food is bound to animal proteins, and first must be freed. To split the B$_{12}$ and the protein apart,

---

* In fact, as we'll explain later, several plants that some supplement manufacturers claim are high in B$_{12}$, such as spirulina and tempeh, actually contain "pseudo-B$_{12}$" analogues that block the uptake of the real vitamin, sometimes causing dangerous deficiencies.

your body uses an enzyme called *pepsin*, which can be produced in sufficient amounts only if there is enough *hydrochloric acid* available in your stomach.

2. Your stomach also produces *intrinsic factor (IF)*, a protein that makes its way into your intestine to be available for a later step in the B_{12} pathway.

3. Next, other proteins called *R-binders* ferry the B_{12} into your small intestine.

4. In the intestine, *intrinsic factor* latches onto the B_{12} (with the help of enzymes called *pancreatic proteases*) and carries it to the last section of the small intestine, the ileum. The cells that line the ileum contain *receptors* that grab onto the B_{12}-IF complex, pulling it into the bloodstream.

5. In the bloodstream, another protein, *transcobalamin II*, carries vitamin B_{12} to the various cells of the body, and then transports the excess to the liver for storage.

This complicated B_{12} metabolism process, far more complex than that for any other vitamin, can break down at any point. The most famous (but not the most common) breakdown in this process is pernicious anemia (an autoimmune disease), a hereditary disorder that once subjected its sufferers to physical and mental deterioration and eventually a terrible death. The disease occurs when the body fails to produce intrinsic factor, making the B_{12} in the diet useless. In 1926, two doctors, George Richards Minot and William Parry Murphy, discovered that feeding half a pound of liver per day to their patients with pernicious anemia dramatically reversed their symptoms.** The physicians, along with George Hoyt Whipple (who had earlier found that liver reversed pernicious anemia symptoms in dogs), won the 1934 Nobel Prize in medicine for their life-saving discovery.***

**Most of the people categorized as having pernicious anemia during this era may have actually suffered from other, more common, forms of B_{12} deficiency. Fortunately, the "liver cure" also worked for many people with acquired forms of B_{12} deficiency.

***Frieda Robshneit-Robbings, together with Whipple, discovered that a diet containing large amounts of liver cured anemia in dogs. Although she coauthored many papers with Whipple, he alone received the Nobel Prize for their joint work.

A far more common cause of B$_{12}$ deficiency, especially in people over fifty, is a condition called *atrophic gastritis*, an inflammation and deterioration of the stomach lining. Atrophic gastritis reduces the secretion of the stomach acid that is needed to separate vitamin B$_{12}$ from protein—a problem often made worse by antacids or other medications (see Chapter 2). In addition, older people have smaller numbers of the cells that produce intrinsic factor.

It's not just the elderly, however, who are at risk. People of any age who undergo gastric surgery for weight loss (gastric bypass), or have partial or complete stomach resections for other reasons, are also candidates for B$_{12}$ deficiency. This is because they lose the cells that produce hydrochloric acid and intrinsic factor. Intestinal surgery involving partial or complete removal of the ileum will also cause B$_{12}$ deficiency, because receptors needed for the absorption of B$_{12}$ are located in this area.

In addition, gastrointestinal disorders such as Crohn's disease (an inflammatory intestinal disease), enteritis, "blind loop" syndrome, or celiac disease can interfere with the absorption of B$_{12}$ even if it's broken down correctly by the body. So can alcohol and many medications, ranging from ulcer drugs to diabetes medications. Exposure to nitrous oxide, either during surgery (including dental surgery) or through recreational drug abuse, can inactivate B$_{12}$. Toxins such as mercury interfere with B$_{12}$'s ability to cross the blood–brain barrier and reach the neurons where it's needed. And, a variety of inborn errors of B$_{12}$ metabolism, which we'll discuss in later chapters, can interfere with B$_{12}$ metabolism at any step from beginning to end.

This is why people who say, "I can't be deficient—I take a vitamin pill every day" are wrong. People who can't metabolize B$_{12}$ from food often can't make use of it efficiently in pill form either, so supplements won't guarantee that you're safe. And, if you're already B$_{12}$-deficient, the few micrograms of B$_{12}$ you'll get from a standard supplement will do as little good as trying to fill an empty swimming pool with a teaspoon of water each day. A person with B$_{12}$ deficiency needs thousands, not just tens or hundreds, of micrograms of B$_{12}$ every day—and in some cases, even people taking thousands of micrograms of oral B$_{12}$ may benefit more by being treated with injections. Moreover, since B$_{12}$ symptoms eventually become irreversible, it's important to treat the problem quickly and aggressively—something you can't do with a handful of pills.

Why is B_{12} deficiency epidemic?

Given the dangers of B_{12} deficiency, it would be natural to assume that doctors put the disorder high on their list of suspects when they see patients with weakness, dizziness, nerve pain or numbness, mental illness, dementia, multiple sclerosis-like symptoms, chronic fatigue, infertility, or other medical problems that can stem from B_{12} deficiency. You'd probably guess, too, that they automatically screen children with unexplained developmental delays or failure to thrive, to determine if B_{12} deficiency is to blame. And you'd assume that they routinely screen patients in the highest-risk age group of sixty and over—and especially patients with unexplained Alzheimer's-like symptoms.

These assumptions, however, are wrong. In reality, most doctors frequently fail to diagnose people with B_{12} deficiency, mistakenly ascribing their symptoms to pre-existing conditions, other diseases, aging, heavy drinking (even when patients deny this), or mental illness—and the results can be catastrophic.

A few years ago, a fifty-four-year-old woman named Rebecca arrived at the hospital in a near-coma, after suffering a fall. The description on her chart was "unresponsive"—but an equally accurate description would be "victim of an unresponsive medical system."

Why? Because throughout Rebecca's life, her body offered up clue after clue of her B_{12} deficiency, but no one noticed. Her mother died at an early age of stomach cancer, a rare cancer in the Western world, but one that often targets people with pernicious anemia. Three of Rebecca's children died shortly after birth—also a red flag for B_{12} deficiency. Rebecca received numerous blood transfusions over the years for anemia, but her doctors never discovered the cause of that anemia. She'd undergone a complete hysterectomy at a relatively early age, possibly as a result of abnormal cells in the cervix and uterus—also a phenomenon that can occur in B_{12}-deficient women. In middle age, she'd begun experiencing excruciating headaches, and she complained of left-side weakness and pains in her arms and legs. She also found it increasingly hard to walk because of her worsening dizziness, and she frequently fell. (The subdural hematoma—bleeding between the brain and the brain's lining—that doctors detected in the emergency room resulted from a fall in which she'd struck her head hard on the door of her truck.) In recent months, *according to her daughter, Rebecca's memory and personality had changed. All of these problems—weakness, leg and arm pains, dizziness, loss of balance, mental changes—are classic symptoms that can occur when B$_{12}$ deficiency progressively damages the brain and nervous system.*

The proximate cause of Rebecca's near-coma when she arrived in the emergency department was a subdural hematoma resulting from hitting her head in repeated falls. The real cause, however, was the dizziness and weakness that made her fall—problems that stemmed directly from her B$_{12}$ deficiency.

Rebecca was severely anemic and required multiple blood transfusions. Her serum B$_{12}$ level was very low, and her red blood cells were very enlarged. (You'll remember that enlarged red blood cells are a classic sign of B$_{12}$ deficiency.) In addition, her platelets were dangerously low, which made it difficult for her blood to clot.

Doctors diagnosed Rebecca with pernicious anemia and a subdural hematoma. Before giving her blood transfusions, they ordered more sensitive tests for B$_{12}$ deficiency. (These tests measure levels of methylmalonic acid and homocysteine, explained later in this book). The test results came back several days later, and were grossly abnormal. Rebecca survived emergency brain surgery, but her hematoma enlarged dangerously afterward, and as a result of the ensuing damage to her brain, she is now in a vegetative state and will never recover.

Rebecca's descent into a permanent coma, at the age of only fifty-four, is a tragedy. But it's only one in a string of tragedies resulting from her misdiagnosis. Rebecca lost years of her life to debilitating vitamin B$_{12}$ deficiency, and it's a virtual certainty that all three of her babies who died at birth or in infancy were victims of her disorder, because Rebecca's depleted stores couldn't nourish them during pregnancy or breast-feeding. (The babies, too, may have suffered from an inherited—and easily detectable and treatable—form of B$_{12}$ deficiency [see Chapter 6].) Even though today's accurate tests weren't available when Rebecca was young, simple serum B$_{12}$ tests would most likely have uncovered her problem, and monthly shots would have prevented the damage her body suffered for decades. Almost undoubtedly, a correct diagnosis also would have saved the lives of Rebecca's babies. But nobody ordered the tests, because none of the physicians Rebecca encountered throughout her life were knowledgeable about vitamin B$_{12}$ deficiency or the inborn errors of B$_{12}$ metabolism.

As medical professionals, we see cases like Rebecca's on a regular basis. Most of the patients with undiagnosed B_{12} deficiency that we encounter aren't at death's door, but the majority have suffered terribly, both physically and emotionally, from symptoms that are destroying their quality of life.

How can something as simple as a vitamin deficiency cause so much suffering? One explanation is that doctors receive surprisingly little training, much of it outdated, in the diagnosis and prevention of B_{12} deficiency.

In general, doctors are trained to recognize only the *blood* abnormalities associated with B_{12} deficiency. In particular, they're trained to look for evidence of *macrocytosis*, or the presence of large, immature red blood cells, a classic sign of B_{12} deficiency anemia. (Anemia, which causes extreme fatigue and weakness, occurs when your red blood cells don't have enough hemoglobin—the substance that ferries oxygen throughout your body. "Macrocytic" or "megaloblastic" anemia, in which the red blood cells are enlarged, stems from too little B_{12} or folic acid.) In addition, many doctors who treat severely anemic patients give these patients blood transfusions *before* ordering sensitive tests to rule out underlying B_{12} deficiency. When doctors order these tests later, the healthy donor blood may mask the abnormalities in the patient's blood.

Doctors who look only for classic blood abnormalities (macrocytic anemia) can misdiagnose the *neurological* abnormalities that stem from B_{12} deficiency, including tingling or "pins and needles" sensations in the hands and feet, memory loss, depression, personality changes, dizziness and loss of balance, or even outright dementia. These nervous system symptoms often precede classic blood abnormalities by many years—and the neurologic damage that underlies them can be permanent by the time tests for the blood abnormalities traditionally associated with B_{12} deficiency begin to come back abnormal.

Many doctors also fail to recognize that high levels of another B vitamin, folic acid (folate), can make the complete blood count (CBC) test results appear normal even when a B_{12} deficiency exists. In 1998, new government rules mandated the fortification of grains with folic acid, increasing the likelihood of missing B_{12} deficiency due to high folate levels which normalize the size of blood cells that otherwise would appear enlarged. Enriching foods with folic acid is a good idea, because it helps prevent spina bifida and related birth defects linked to low folic acid levels—but ironically, the same enrichment that protects many babies from harm also endangers other babies and adults whose doctors rely solely on traditional blood tests to detect B$_{12}$ deficiency.

Still another factor contributing powerfully to the rampant non-diagnosis of B$_{12}$ deficiency—indeed, possibly the most important factor—is money. B$_{12}$ deficiency mimics many other diseases, so your doctor can't know if you're low in B$_{12}$ simply by analyzing your symptoms. Also, your doctor can't determine if you're deficient or not simply by

Types of Tests for B$_{12}$ Deficiency

Serum Vitamin B$_{12}$ Test

Measures the level of vitamin B$_{12}$ in your blood serum. Often gives false positive or false negative values, and is less sensitive and less specific than the MMA test described below. Also, there is much controversy as to what constitutes a normal result for this test, with many experts believing that the current level is far too low. Because of its limitations, this test should be used in conjunction with the MMA.

Methylmalonic Acid (MMA) Test

Measures the amount of MMA in the urine or blood. Elevated levels of MMA indicate B$_{12}$ deficiency (see Chapter 11). The most accurate test for B$_{12}$ deficiency is the urinary MMA/creatinine ratio test developed in 1985. MMA is 40 times more concentrated in the urine than in the blood, and the urinary MMA test does not produce false positives or false negatives as can occur with the serum MMA. The urinary MMA is needed to confirm or rule out B$_{12}$ deficiency.

Homocysteine (Hcy) test

Measures the level of homocysteine in the plasma. Elevated levels of Hcy can indicate vitamin B$_{12}$, vitamin B$_6$, or folate deficiency. Hcy may also be elevated in a few other medical conditions (see Chapter 11). The Hcy test is not necessary to diagnose B$_{12}$ deficiency, but is a valuable adjunct to the MMA and serum B$_{12}$ tests. The higher your Hcy level, the higher your risk of cardiovascular disease (see Chapter 5).

(See "Reference Ranges for Diagnostic Tests" on the next page for ranges considered acceptable for these tests.)

Reference Ranges for Diagnostic Tests

Serum B12:   211 – 911 pg/ml (155 – 670 pmol/L)
              180 – 914 pg/ml (132 – 672 pmol/L)

Urinary MMA: < 3.8 µg MMA/mg creatinine
             (3.6 µmole/mmole creatinine)

Normal Serum MMA:
         0.07 (some labs use 0.04) – 0.27 µmol/L
         or 70 – 270 nmol/L

Plasma Homocysteine: 4.0 – 12.0 µmol/L

1. Ranges for the serum B_{12} test vary among different laboratories. Experts believe serum B_{12} levels below 350 pg/ml warrant further testing.

2. Falsely high values have not been reported for the urinary MMA test. This is because the urinary MMA test is normalized to urine creatinine, which corrects for dehydration and kidney problems. This is why we recommend the urinary MMA for screening.

3. Even though some laboratories use the range of < 0.4 µmol/L for normal serum MMA, a mild B_{12} deficiency can be present with serum MMA values > 0.27 µmol/L. Therefore, patients with borderline values must be monitored and retested within six months, or treated if the patient is symptomatic. If B_{12} therapy is started, patients should be evaluated for changes in hematologic signs, lowering of MMA, or improvement of symptoms. Again, because false positive results can occur with the serum MMA, we recommend the urinary MMA.

(See Chapter 11 for possible causes of false positive and false negative results of serum B_{12}, serum MMA, and plasma Hcy.)

ordering an inexpensive serum B$_{12}$ test or a blood smear (a test for the enlarged red blood cells and abnormal white blood cells [neutrophils] seen in clear-cut cases of B$_{12}$ deficiency anemia). These tests will uncover many cases of B$_{12}$ deficiency, but it's possible to have a nearly fatal deficiency and still have normal lab results. To confirm or rule out a problem with your B$_{12}$ levels, your doctor needs to order a more sophisticated test which measures the amount of methylmalonic acid in the urine. (See chart on page 10 for a brief description of the tests discussed in this book. Chapters 10 and 11 offer a more in-depth explanation.)

The urinary MMA test described in the chart costs insurance companies or patients less than $100, which isn't much money—especially when you compare it to thousands of dollars for CT scans, MRIs, and other tests that doctors routinely order. Moreover, the tests are virtually always covered by insurance, but not all doctors know this. The unfortunate result of this lack of awareness is that many physicians forgo these tests, thus condemning patients to a lifetime of suffering.

Ironically, this misplaced concern over the expense of B$_{12}$ testing costs the medical system far more than it saves, because B$_{12}$ deficiency is remarkably simple to detect and even easier to treat. Patients treated in the early stages of the disease usually experience complete recovery, with even severe symptoms such as vision loss, agonizing leg pains, paralysis, multiple sclerosis-like symptoms, psychosis, and dementia often receding in months or even weeks. Moreover, unlike many medical problems, B$_{12}$ deficiency is very inexpensive to treat. Monthly B$_{12}$ shots are about $1.25 each, meaning that the cost of treating B$_{12}$ deficiency, once it's identified, is *about $15.00 per year*. Compare this to the cost of giving a depressed patient, with undiagnosed B$_{12}$ deficiency, unnecessary antidepressants, which can be as high as $1,000 a year—or to the cost of caring for a B$_{12}$ deficient patient misdiagnosed as having Alzheimer's, multiple sclerosis, or mental retardation, an expense that can run $50,000 a year or more, for decades.

The cost in human terms, of course, is far greater. There is no price one can place on the pain of individuals whose undiagnosed B$_{12}$ deficiency leads to severe, irreversible physical and mental disability.

In 2000, a fifty-year-old Illinois woman, Vicki Lambert, received a $3 million out-of-court settlement from two hospitals and two physician groups. Lambert charged doctors at each of these institutions failed to *diagnose her B_{12} deficiency, leaving her permanently crippled. She suffers from chronic painful neuropathy, uses specialized crutches to walk, and has irreversible cognitive deficits. She is unable to work as a nurse because of her disability and has moved to a one-story home because she could no longer go up and down stairs.*

"Unless someone were in my shoes, you can't imagine," Lambert told a newspaper reporter. "I remember lying in bed and feeling death would be better because I was so sick."[5]

In a similar 1999 case, a sixty-four-year-old Georgia woman was awarded $3.1 million after a missed diagnosis of B_{12} deficiency. The woman now requires a wheelchair as a result of permanent nerve damage due to her doctors' failure to identify her condidtion.[6]

How B_{12} deficiency attacks the body

As you can guess from the cases we described at the start of this chapter, it's impossible to paint a simple picture of what B_{12} deficiency looks like. When B_{12} deficiency attacks the body, it takes many guises, depending in part on the age and genetic vulnerabilities of its victims, and the length and severity of the deficiency. Also, because B_{12} deficiency is progressive, signs and symptoms may take years to develop. The following list outlines signs and symptoms that can stem from B_{12} deficiency.

Note: If you have any of the following signs or symptoms, it does not necessarily mean that you have a B_{12} deficiency. These symptoms can stem from many causes. However, it does mean that your doctor needs to rule out B_{12} deficiency as a possible culprit.

Mental changes
- irritability
- apathy
- sleepiness
- suspiciousness (paranoia)
- personality changes
- depression (including postpartum depression)
- memory loss
- dementia, intellectual deterioration
- hallucinations

• violent behavior
• in children, developmental delay and/or autistic behavior

Neurological signs and symptoms
• abnormal sensations (pain, tingling and/or numbness of legs, arms, trunk, or other area)
• diminished sense of touch, pain, and/or temperature
• loss of position sense (awareness of body position)
• weakness (legs, arms, trunk, or other area)
• clumsiness (stiff or awkward movements)
• tremor
• symptoms mimicking Parkinson's disease or multiple sclerosis
• spasticity of muscles
• incontinence (urine and/or stool)
• paralysis
• vision changes (decreased vision or loss of vision)
• damage to the optic nerve (optic neuritis, inflammation, or atrophy of the optic nerve)

Vascular problems
• transient ischemic attacks (TIAs, or "mini-strokes")
• cerebral vascular accident (CVA or "stroke")
• coronary artery disease
• myocardial infarction ("heart attack")
• congestive heart failure
• palpitations
• orthostatic hypotension (low blood pressure when standing, which can cause fainting and falls)
• deep vein thrombosis (blood clot to the leg or arm)
• pulmonary embolism (blood clot to the lung)

Additional signs and symptoms
• shortness of breath
• generalized weakness
• chronic fatigue or tiredness
• loss of appetite/weight loss or anorexia
• epigastric pain (poor digestion, full or bloated feeling after eating small or normal sized meals)

- gastrointestinal problems (diarrhea, constipation)
- osteoporosis
- increased susceptibility to infection
- in newborns and infants, failure to thrive
- tinnitus (ringing or roaring in the ears)
- vitiligo (white patches of skin) or, conversely, hyperpigmentation of skin
- prematurely gray hair

It amazes many people that a single medical problem—B_{12} deficiency—can cause so many medical symptoms. But the reason is simple: B_{12} wears many hats, playing key roles in the health of your nerves, your blood, and your immune system, as well as in the formation of DNA (the molecular blueprint for making the substances that create and maintain your body). Thus, B_{12} deficiency can impair the functioning of almost any part of your body.

In particular, B_{12} deficiency often strikes the nervous system, causing damage to the soft fatty material called *myelin* that surrounds and protects nerve fibers. This damage *(demyelination)*, which can be compared to the fraying of an electrical wire, can cause you to develop mysterious and frightening neurological problems, ranging from numb, tingling, or painful legs and arms, to loss of balance, vision loss, impotence, or incontinence. Because your brain and nervous system control your mental state, the demyelination caused by B_{12} deficiency can also lead to memory loss, "fuzzy" thinking, personality changes, depression, or even psychosis or dementia. (In a child, the damage can be even worse, because the young brain is still forming and requires adequate B_{12} to grow normally.)

As B_{12} deficiency continues, your immune system also falls prey, because it can no longer produce enough disease-fighting white blood cells. Thus, you become an easier target for viral or bacterial infections. Your gastrointestinal system suffers as well, because your body can't make enough cells to replace your intestinal lining efficiently, so you may experience diarrhea, nausea, or severe appetite loss—all of which can worsen your B_{12} deficiency. And eventually, as your B_{12} deficit grows, you're likely to feel exhausted and weak due to the anemia that occurs when your body can't make enough healthy blood cells to carry oxygen to the cells of your body.

At the same time, B$_{12}$ deficiency causes a breakdown in a crucial metabolic pathway that detoxifies the potentially dangerous amino acid homocysteine. As homocysteine accumulates in your blood, it dramatically increases your risk of coronary artery disease, stroke, and blood clots. If you become pregnant, high homocysteine levels will also make you more vulnerable to preeclampsia, a potentially fatal pregnancy complication.

If you're a woman, the blood abnormalities resulting from B$_{12}$ defi-

---

Systems Affected by Vitamin B$_{12}$ Deficiency

Neurologic

pain, numbness, "pins and needles" sensations, balance problems, falling, weakness, paralysis, confusion, dementia, depression, psychosis, incontinence, vision loss

Hematologic (blood)

fatigue, weakness, anemia, enlarged spleen or liver, unexplained blood loss, blood transfusions

Immunologic

poor wound healing, increased susceptibility to infections, increased risk of breast cancer

Vascular

coronary artery disease, blood clots in lungs or extremities, mini-stroke, stroke, heart attack

Gastrointestinal

indigestion, malabsorption, abdominal pain, weight loss, constipation, diarrhea, gastric stasis, increased risk of gastric cancer (if B$_{12}$ deficiency is caused by autoimmune pernicious anemia)

Musculoskeletal

fractures from falling due to balance problems; suppressed activity of osteoblasts (cells that build new bone), which contributes to osteoporosis and fractures

Genitourinary

unnecessary repeated Pap smears and GYN procedures (D&C, LEEP), unnecessary hysterectomies, urinary incontinence, impotence, infertility

---

ciency may affect the lining of your uterus and cervix, causing cervical dysplasia (abnormal cervical cell appearance) that can be mistaken for a pre-cancerous condition. But B_{12} deficiency doesn't just mimic cancer warning signs; it also puts you at higher risk for certain cancers, whether you're male or female. Pernicious anemia, the classic form of vitamin B_{12} deficiency, is a strong risk factor for stomach cancer, and there is mounting evidence linking deficient levels of B_{12} to breast cancer, as well.

The bad news... and the good news

So far, what we've told you is frightening. Millions of North Americans suffer from undiagnosed B_{12} deficiency—and you may be one of them. If you are, this disease could be attacking your brain, your cardiovascular system, and your immune system, putting you at risk for everything from Alzheimer's-like dementia to heart disease and cancer. You're not safe even if you get regular checkups, because your doctor may miss the correct diagnosis until it's too late to reverse your symptoms. And if you're a woman who is B_{12} deficient and you don't find out about your condition in time, even your children may suffer permanent damage to their bodies and brains.

That's the bad news. The good news is that if it's caught early, B_{12} deficiency is one of the simplest disorders in the world to treat. In fact, many formerly B_{12}-deficient people say that getting a diagnosis was the best thing that ever happened to them—because it meant that the "incurable" neuropathy, weakness, infertility, MS-like symptoms, depression, or other problems that afflicted them weren't incurable after all. In this book, we'll share the stories of once-bedridden people who can walk again... people freed from excruciating leg and back pain... individuals cured of memory loss, depression, schizophrenic symptoms, and even dementia... people freed from the need for repeated blood transfusions for mysterious anemia... people able to conceive healthy babies after B_{12} treatment... and even developmentally disabled or autistic children who made almost miraculous gains after their deficient B_{12} levels were detected and treated. All of these individuals experienced dramatic improvement after undergoing the simplest and safest of treatments: a few shots (or, in some cases, pills) containing megadoses of vitamin B_{12}. Their stories are a powerful counterpoint to the horrific stories of patients who have suffered devastating injuries, years of poor health, or terrible ill-

Who's at Greatest Risk for B$_{12}$ Deficiency?

Anyone, at any age, can become B$_{12}$-deficient. Thus, you need to be tested immediately if you develop any of the symptoms we've described in this chapter. However, certain people are at significantly elevated risk. They include the following:

• Vegetarians and vegans

• People aged sixty and over

• People who've undergone any gastric and/or intestinal surgery, including bariatric surgery for weight loss purposes (gastric bypass)

• People who regularly use antacids, metformin and related diabetes drugs, or other medications that can interfere with B$_{12}$ absorption

• People who undergo surgeries or dental procedures involving nitrous oxide, or who abuse this drug recreationally

• People with a history of eating disorders (anorexia or bulimia)

• People with a history of alcoholism

• People with a family history of pernicious anemia

• People diagnosed with anemia (including iron deficiency anemia)

• People with Crohn's disease, irritable bowel syndrome, celiac disease, or any other disease that causes malabsorption of nutrients

• People with autoimmune disorders (especially thyroid disorders such as Hashimoto's thyroiditis and Graves' disease), type 1 diabetes, or a family history of these disorders

• Women with a history of infertility or multiple miscarriages

• Infants born to and/or breast-fed by women who are deficient in B$_{12}$ for any reason

nesses, and who have incurred huge medical expenses as well, due to the non-diagnosis or late diagnosis of their B_{12} deficiency.

We want it to be perfectly clear, at the outset of this book, that B_{12} isn't a "magic bullet." The symptoms we've outlined have many causes, and B_{12} deficiency is only one of them. But patients and doctors need to be aware that B_{12} deficiency often *does* cause these symptoms, and that doctors who fail to rule it out may be condemning millions of patients to unnecessary debility or even death. Conversely, the brief amount of time and money required to identify B_{12} deficiency is a small investment to make—and whether you're a doctor or a medical consumer, it may be the most important investment you'll ever make.

Note: Vitamin B_{12} treatment is quite possibly the safest medical treatment on earth. However, one small group of people—those with a rare disorder called Leber's hereditary optic neuropathy—should never take cyanocobalamin, one specific form of B_{12}. Information about safe forms of B_{12} treatment for these individuals is contained in Chapter 11.

Notes

1. Study cited in "B_{12} deficiency may be more widespread than thought," Judy McBride, Agricultural Research Service website, U.S. Department of Agriculture, August 2, 2000. http://www.ars.usda.gov/is/pr/2000/000802.htm.
2. Shahar, A., Feiglin, L., Shahar, D. R., Levy, S., and Seligsohn, U. High prevalence and impact of subnormal serum vitamin B_{12} levels in Israeli elders admitted to a geriatric hospital. *Journal of Nutrition, Health and Aging* (2001) 5:124–7.
3. Crane, M.G., Register, U. D., Lukens, R. H., and Gregory, R. Cobalamin (CBL). Studies on two total vegetarian (vegan) families. *Vegetarian Nutrition: An International Journal* 1998, 2(3):87–92.
4. Bissoli, L., Di Francesco, V., Ballarin, A., Mandragona, R., Trespidi, R., Brocco, G., Caruso, B., Bosello, O., and Zamboni, M. Effect of vegetarian diet on homocysteine levels. *Annals of Nutrition and Metabolism* 2002, 46(2):73–9.
5. Ordower, G. "Batavia woman mkes appeal to Bush," Daily Herald, January 6, 2005.
6. Www.emarcusdavis.com/practice/practice_hmom.html.

Is It Aging—or Is It B$_{12}$ Deficiency?

*"T*he lack of knowledge about vitamin B$_{12}$ deficiency is astounding, especially when you consider the number of elderly individuals that are afflicted now and, with the graying of society, the number that will soon be at risk."* —Robert Schmidt, M.D., board member, American Society on Aging[1]

Emily came into the emergency department during my shift, bruised and shaken after a frightening fall. X rays revealed a fracture in her right arm, but the tiny, fragile eighty-nine-year-old had more problems than just a broken bone. She seemed confused, made little sense when she talked, and couldn't tell me the date or time. She walked slowly and unsteadily, with a wide-based gait, as though she couldn't tell where her feet were. She looked thin, pale, and malnourished, and she needed to wear Depends because she wet herself.

Emily came to us with a diagnosis of dementia. Luckily for her, the doctor on my shift ordered a serum B$_{12}$ level; it came back 156pg/ml, an indication of deficiency. Her low B$_{12}$ levels could explain every one of her symptoms—the fall, the confusion and memory loss, her abnormal gait, her pallor and incontinence—yet none of her previous doctors had ever checked her B$_{12}$ levels. They just thought she was old.

Being old isn't easy. Being an elderly patient is even harder. That's because the medical profession, like the public in general, tends to stereotype seniors. They're "drifty." They forget things. They fall a lot. They have aches and pains everywhere. They get senile.

But in reality, these problems aren't "normal" or "typical." When we see them in a patient who's twenty, thirty, or forty, we usually search until we find a cause. But when a seventy-year-old complains of forgetfulness, depression, or incontinence, medical professionals too often think to themselves, "That's to be expected when you get old." As a result, vast numbers of seniors suffer unnecessarily from problems that go undiagnosed and untreated—frequent falls, difficulty in walking, memory lapses, depression, and crippling aches and pains—simply because we fail to look for their causes.

If we do take note of these problems, all too often, we simply say, "It's just a new symptom of your existing medical conditions." We blame leg pains on diabetes or arthritis, and falls on failing vision or poor reflexes. We dismiss depression as a normal response to losing a spouse or friends, and we say that memory lapses are simply part of the aging process. But when we dismiss aging patients' suffering as "normal," we consign many of these patients to nursing homes, or even to death, when they have treatable problems. And one common problem in people over sixty is vitamin B$_{12}$ deficiency.

Seniors are a high-risk group for severe B$_{12}$ deficiency for several reasons. One is that 30 to 40 percent of them develop a condition called *atrophic gastritis*, or inflammation and wasting of the stomach lining. This drastically decreases their levels of stomach acid, which is needed to free B$_{12}$ from animal proteins, so that it can be absorbed.

Doctors commonly treat elderly patients' stomach upsets and indigestion with drugs such as Prevacid, Prilosec, Zantac, Pepcid, Aciphex, Nexium, and Protonix, and seniors frequently dose themselves with over-the-counter antacids. Unfortunately, all of these medications reduce stomach acid even further, causing B$_{12}$ levels to drop still further.

In addition, many seniors eat poorly, and those who live on limited budgets often forgo vitamin supplements and meat (the primary dietary source of B$_{12}$) to save pennies. Older individuals frequently lose interest in food, especially if they live alone or if they find it difficult to eat due to indigestion or sore mouths. Many have trouble chewing their food—which again makes them avoid meat—because of bad teeth or poorly fitting dentures. And a high percentage of seniors have a history of gastric or intestinal surgeries, or of radiation treatment for cancers of the abdominal or pelvic organs, either of which can dramatically increase the risk of having dangerously low B$_{12}$ levels.

Some older people actually suffer not from an age-related problem in extracting and absorbing B$_{12}$, but from true pernicious anemia (an autoimmune disease; see Chapter 1) that has gone undiagnosed for decades. One case we witnessed involved a seventy-seven-year-old woman with symptoms so advanced that she'd been placed under hospice care. Doctors had misdiagnosed her increasing motor problems for many years, eventually labeling them as "multiple sclerosis," when she was seventy-two years old.

When seniors start showing symptoms of B$_{12}$ deficiency, their doctors often mask these symptoms with drugs—Detrol for incontinence; Aricept or Namenda for Alzheimer's-like deterioration; Haldol or Risperdal for psychotic behavior; Prozac, Zoloft, Effexor, or Serzone for depression; Paxil, Xanax, or Ativan for anxiety—without ever determining their cause. This makes patients feel better, but not for long. That's because the damage caused by the deficiency is still eating away at these patients' brains, nervous systems, and cardiovascular systems.

It's ironic that in the name of cost containment, the usual reason for failing to order B$_{12}$ tests, doctors often prescribe expensive drugs to treat symptoms that could—in cases where these symptoms stem from B$_{12}$ deficiency—be eliminated by B$_{12}$ shots costing about fifteen dollars a year. Compare this cost to more than $2,200 a year for Cognex, often prescribed for patients with dementia due to undiagnosed B$_{12}$ deficiency— or to the $1,000-per-year tab for the drug Neurontin, often used to treat numbness and leg pains that can stem from deficient stores of B$_{12}$. These drugs are "penny wise and pound foolish" for another reason: They often allow symptoms to progress, undiagnosed and untreated, to the point where patients need expensive hospital or nursing home care.

A problem of epidemic proportions

How many seniors suffer or die because B$_{12}$ deficiency impairs their minds and wreaks havoc on their hearts, blood vessels, and nervous and immune systems? The data we've seen indicate that there are millions—enough to have a huge impact on medical care expenses in the United States, and to touch almost every family in some way. As we noted in the last chapter, between 15 and 40 percent of people over sixty have low serum B$_{12}$ levels. This means that at least one in seven people over sixty—and possibly as many as four in ten—are at risk of suffering from nerve, brain, heart, and blood vessel damage caused by an often "silent" deficiency.

Common Drugs that Can Put Seniors at Risk for B$_{12}$ Deficiency

The following drugs impair absorption of B$_{12}$ in various ways (see Chapter 10 for a more detailed explanation). Seniors who take these medications regularly, or take a combination of them, are at increased risk of developing B$_{12}$ deficiency:

Drug	Reason for use
Prevacid, Prilosec, Protonix, Nexium, Aciphex...	Heartburn GERD (acid reflux) Ulcers H. Pylori infection
Zantac, Tagamet, Axid, Pepcid...	Heartburn GERD Ulcers Upper GI bleeding
Alternagel, Maalox, MOM, Mylanta, Riopan, Tums...	Heartburn Acid indigestion Peptic ulcer disease GERD Gastritis Hiatal hernia
Glucophage, Glucovance...	Diabetes
K-Lor, K-Lyte, Klotrix, K-Dur, Micro-K, Slow-K, potassium chloride...	Potassium deficiency—often prescribed for patients with congestive heart failure, kidney failure, or cirrhosis, of the liver, and for patients who receive diuretics ("water pills," such as Lasix, Bumex, and hydrochlorothiazide [HCTZ])
Colchicine...	Gout
Questran...	Elevated cholesterol levels
Neomycin...	Infections
Para-aminosalicylic acid...	Tuberculosis

Common Drugs that Can Mask Undiagnosed B$_{12}$ Deficiency

Doctors who prescribe the following drugs to treat B$_{12}$-deficient patients' symptoms, without uncovering the cause of those symptoms, can allow undetected B$_{12}$ deficiency to progress to incurable or even life-threatening stages:

Drug	Can mask these signs and symptoms that frequently stem from B$_{12}$ deficiency in the elderly
Celexa, Effexor, Elavil, Nardil, Pamelor, Paxil, Prozac, Serzone, Sinequon, Tofranil, Wellbutrin, Zoloft...	Depression
Ativan, Klonopin, Librium, Paxil, Serax, Tranxene, Valium, Xanax...	Anxiety and panic disorder
Viagra, Cialis, Levitra...	Erectile dysfunction
Aricept, Cognex, Exelon, Reminyl...	Dementia
Antivert...	Dizziness, imbalance, and vertigo
Detrol, Ditropan, Levbid...	Incontinence
Compazine, Geodon, Haldol, Navane, Risperdal, Stelazine, Tegretol, Thorazine...	Psychosis
Ambien, Dalmane, Halcion, Restoril...	Insomnia
Cylert, Ritalin...	Fatigue
Diamox, Inderal, Mysoline, Symmetrel...	Tremors
Elavil, Neurontin, Tegretol...	Numbness and tingling
Folic acid (folate), Folvite, Apo-Folic (folate is a nutrient often given to alcoholics and patients with poor diets, and also used to lower the risk of colon cancer or to treat high homocysteine levels)...	Blood abnormalities (enlarged red blood cells)

In 1996, Dr. Ralph Carmel, an expert on B$_{12}$ deficiency, estimated that more than 800,000 people in the United States over the age of sixty had undiagnosed and untreated pernicious anemia.[2] This is only the tip of the iceberg when it comes to B$_{12}$ deficiency, because the number of seniors with deficiency due to poor diet or malabsorption problems is believed to be significantly greater than the number of people with pernicious anemia.

Furthermore, the number of new cases of B$_{12}$ deficiency is rising each year as the senior population grows. In 1993, Dr. Eric Norman used the highly accurate urinary MMA test to re-evaluate 299 independently living seniors aged sixty-five and older whose screenings for B$_{12}$ deficiency had been normal approximately one year earlier. The re-testing showed that more than 2 percent had developed B$_{12}$ deficiency over the year. "Thus," Dr. Norman says, "for the thirty million United States elderly, 600,000 new cases per year are possible."[3] His findings strongly indicate that yearly urinary MMA screening is warranted for the elderly population.

Yet only a small percentage of seniors will be sent for even a rudimentary serum B$_{12}$ test, and almost none will receive the more sophisticated urinary MMA test needed to rule out B$_{12}$ deficiency. As a result, many will wind up wheelchair-bound or bedridden, suffer unnecessary strokes or heart disease, or even develop irreversible dementia.

Why is this obvious diagnosis so often missed in older patients? There are a number of reasons, involving time pressures, stereotypes about the elderly, and concerns about money. The following are the excuses we hear most often from our colleagues:

1. *"They're just old."* As we've noted, far too many medical professionals equate old age with decrepitude. As a result, they don't spend the time and effort it takes to determine whether an elderly person's leg pains, difficulty in walking, falls, confusion, memory loss, or other symptoms are "just old age," or stem from treatable B$_{12}$ deficiency.

2. *"We can't screen for everything."* The doctors who say this are unaware of the high rate of B$_{12}$ deficiency in older patients, as compared to the rates of other problems for which they routinely screen. At one hospital we studied, for instance, 316,000 patients used the laboratory's services in 1999, but doctors screened only 121 patients for B$_{12}$ deficiency. Therefore, doctors ordered B$_{12}$ tests for only one of every 2,612

patients (0.04 percent) using the facility's laboratory services. Yet, as we noted, a minimum of 15 percent of people over the age of sixty, and potentially as many as 40 percent, have deficient or borderline B$_{12}$ levels. (In contrast, this hospital ordered more than 600 serum calcium tests *per week*, even though only about 10 percent of patients had abnormal serum calcium levels.)

3. *"It's someone else's job."* Elderly patients often have a primary care doctor and a host of specialists, and these doctors frequently assume that another physician will check for B$_{12}$ deficiency. The emergency room doctor assumes that it's the primary care doctor's responsibility. The primary care doctor assumes that it's the cardiologist's or endocrinologist's or surgeon's or neurologist's problem. And all too often, nobody follows through.

4. *"His last doctor probably checked it."* Under managed care, seniors often get shuffled from plan to plan, and from doctor to doctor. Each new doctor may assume—usually incorrectly—that a previous physician did a B$_{12}$ level.

5. *"A serum B$_{12}$ is good enough."* As we explained in Chapter 1, a serum B$_{12}$ *isn't* good enough, by a long shot. Many seniors with borderline or perfectly normal serum B$_{12}$ levels are severely deficient, some to the point of developing Alzheimer's-like dementia.

Sadly, this is not common knowledge in the medical community. If the serum B$_{12}$ is in the ballpark, and a blood smear doesn't show any gross abnormalities, many doctors think they've ruled out B$_{12}$ deficiency. Yet in most seniors, neurological abnormalities precede blood abnormalities by years.

How widespread is ignorance about the need for additional tests to rule out low B$_{12}$? As we noted earlier, one test that's necessary is the urinary MMA. In the study mentioned above, which we conducted at a hospital that treated tens of thousands of elderly patients and had a total of 316,000 patients of all ages using laboratory services in 1999, doctors ordered the serum MMA test to rule out B$_{12}$ deficiency only twenty-nine times during the entire year. This means that only one out of every 10,897 patients, or 0.01 percent of all patients, were more adequately screened to diagnose or rule out B$_{12}$ deficiency that year. No urinary MMAs, however, were performed.

6. *"I already have a logical explanation for her symptoms."* Elderly patients often have one or more pre-existing diseases, and it's easy to dismiss new symptoms as part of an existing medical problem.

For instance, I recently talked to a once-active man who began suffering years ago, at the age of sixty-eight, from foot and leg numbness. He's now barely able to walk far enough to do a little grocery shopping, and he's dangerous when he drives, because he can't feel his feet. For a decade, every doctor he saw assumed that his symptoms were side effects of diabetes. But given his age, his poor eating habits, and his history of iron-deficiency anemia and hospitalization for a "massive blood loss" that couldn't be explained,* I knew that his symptoms were also quite likely to be due to B$_{12}$ deficiency. Yet despite the fact that he'd seen fifteen doctors in the past two years alone, he'd never been tested.

Why does it matter? Because if the numbness stems from B$_{12}$ deficiency, it's treatable, at least in its early stages. If it stems from diabetes, it usually isn't. It might not make a difference to the doctor, but it makes all of the difference in the world to a patient who wants to continue to enjoy driving, shopping, and living independently. Moreover, the neuropathy due to B$_{12}$ deficiency is just one step in a process that, left uncorrected, is likely to become a long slide into severe debility, or even death. The man I just described was saved from this fate because he took my advice, got tested, and found out that he is indeed B$_{12}$-deficient. It may be too late to reverse his leg pain and numbness, but it's not too late to save him from the psychosis or dementia that chronically depleted B$_{12}$ levels can cause.

Blaming a patient's problems on a single condition also overlooks the fact that many older patients' problems are multifactorial; in other words, they have more than one cause. Even if a patient's symptoms can be linked to diabetes or Parkinson's disease or another known condition, a B$_{12}$ deficiency may very well be contributing to these symptoms. Identifying one disorder is no justification for ignoring another. (As an old medical saying goes, "If a patient has six nails in his foot, and you remove one, he still has a sore foot.")

7. *"The insurance company isn't going to pay for this."* This is a common response, in a cost-cutting era in which every test comes under scrutiny. We have two answers for doctors who are concerned about the

---

*B$_{12}$ deficiency can cause severe anemia, requiring blood transfusions. Doctors typically equate severe anemia with internal bleeding and fail to order B$_{12}$ and iron studies before giving transfusions. Testing patients for B$_{12}$ and iron status after blood transfusions are given yields inaccurate results, clouding the clinical picture.

financial aspects of B$_{12}$ testing. One is that when they code for B$_{12}$ tests correctly (see Appendix S), insurers will cover them. The other is, "Would your patient think it's worth around $70—the cost of a urinary MMA— to prevent a stroke, congestive heart failure, a crippling fall, chronic disability, or dementia?"

We guarantee that patients would say yes. So would doctors and insurers, if they realized that they could save the health care and insurance industries enormous amounts of money by diagnosing B$_{12}$ deficiency before it causes expensive, chronic illnesses. Dr. Eric Norman, the biochemist who developed the urinary MMA test for B$_{12}$ deficiency in 1985, says that widescale identification and treatment of B$_{12}$ deficiency would "help seniors maintain their productivity, dignity, and independence while saving billions of dollars annually in health care costs."[4]

The long darkness: when low B$_{12}$ destroys the mind

The first time you forget your best friend's name, you laugh and write it off as a "senior moment." But the moments start happening more and more often.

You drive to the grocery store and can't remember where you parked. You forget to pay the electric bill three months in a row. You set out for the doctor's office and wind up miles away, not sure how you got there. As time passes, you find yourself unable to add a simple column of numbers or address a birthday card. Familiar people begin to look like strangers, and the crossword puzzles you once loved become a meaningless blur of words. You forget what day it is, where you live, what your children's names are. You begin wetting yourself, and one winter morning the neighbors find you outside in your underwear. You become angry, frightened, and confused.

Your daughter cries when your doctor says you need to be moved to a long-term care facility. Soon, you find yourself living in a tiny room, being led to cafeteria meals by people you don't know. Eventually, the same people need to dress you, bathe you, and help you go to the bathroom, because you can no longer care for yourself. You don't know why you're there. You don't know what's become of your home, your family, and your life. In time, you don't even know who you are.

This is the tragic pattern of dementia, a relentless decline in memory and mental ability. Striking more than five million Americans, dementia turns victims' "golden years" into years of torment, devastates families emotionally and financially, transforms loving spouses and children into exhausted full-time caretakers, and fills America's nursing homes with sad, bewildered patients with no hope of recovery.

If you're dealing with someone suffering from dementia, you know the pain of watching a vibrant individual become a different person— one who becomes agitated, inconsolably sad, paranoid, or even violent or hateful. You know the agony of watching a friend or relative stare at you vacantly, wondering who you are. And you know the guilt of hoping for a loved one to die, because dying is preferable to the slow and inexorable loss of self that dementia causes.

But what you may not know is that *dementia isn't always incurable—even when doctors say it is.* As neurologist Sydney Walker III, M.D., noted, "Many patients do suffer from Alzheimer's and other dementias; but [many others], who are labeled as having dementia, are actually suffering from problems that can be corrected. Studies suggest, in fact, that up to 60 percent of patients tentatively labeled as having 'dementia' actually have treatable and reversible disorders."[5] There are millions of people with true dementias, such as Alzheimer's disease and Pick's dementia (although even Alzheimer's may be linked to B$_{12}$—see later in this chapter), but for each of them it's likely that there's another "demented" patient with a disorder that's treatable and curable. And in many cases, that disorder is B$_{12}$ deficiency.

If you review the statistics we've already cited, this isn't surprising. Remember that

- Up to 15 percent of seniors, and up to 40 percent of symptomatic people over sixty, have low or borderline B$_{12}$ levels.
- The symptoms of B$_{12}$ deficiency can include confusion, memory loss, personality changes, paranoia, depression, and other behaviors that look just like incurable dementia. Dementia stemming from B$_{12}$ deficiency also mimics other dementias in its progress, which usually is gradual but relentless. Thus, it's all too easy to mistakenly write off B$_{12}$-deficiency dementia as incurable.
- There is no test that can diagnose Alzheimer's conclusively in a living patient. Thus, the only way to differentiate between Alzheimer's and other causes of dementia is to rule

out all other causes—something that's too rarely done. (A recent study in Finland, a country with a highly advanced medical system that is comparable to that of the United States, found that only 20 percent of patients with symptoms of dementia were screened for B$_{12}$ deficiency.[6])

- As we've noted, a serum B$_{12}$ test, which itself is too infrequently ordered for elderly patients, is an inadequate measure of B$_{12}$ status. Thus, while most people over sixty aren't tested at all for B$_{12}$ deficiency, even those who *are* tested usually receive a fairly crude test that can't rule out the disorder. In addition, the B$_{12}$ levels we accept as normal for the elderly may be far too low. Behavioral medicine specialist Dr. Mark Goodman has treated 24 demented patients whose seemingly normal serum B$_{12}$ levels masked a severe B$_{12}$ deficiency. When he gave these patients B$_{12}$ injections, every one of them improved dramatically.[7]

While most doctors are unaware of the prevalence of B$_{12}$ deficiency in patients with symptoms of dementia, the medical literature clearly shows that the problem is not a rare one. One study, for instance, found that one in seven demented patients seen consecutively by a clinic had subnormal serum B$_{12}$ levels.[8] Identifying such patients early is crucial, because prompt treatment in the early phases of B$_{12}$ deficiency can restore patients to normal or near-normal functioning.

In an article in Discover *magazine, Leslie Bernstein, M.D. told of her shock when she saw "Pop," a formerly active, healthy patient of hers. "If his grandson hadn't been holding him up, he'd have pitched straight forward onto his face," she said. "Saliva dribbled from the corners of his mouth. His eyes were vacant." In the span of a single month, Pop had changed from a healthy jogger and loving grandfather into a confused, incontinent man whose doctors diagnosed him as having senile dementia.*

Pop's blood work looked normal, except that his red blood cells were slightly larger than normal. His psychiatrist had concluded that he suffered from "toxic/organic disease without significant depression." Luckily, his family brought him to see Dr. Bernstein, who almost immediately thought of a more logical explanation for Pop's drastic decline:

Due to his age and vegetarian diet, he was probably B$_{12}$-deficient. Dr. Bernstein quickly ordered blood work that showed that Pop had B$_{12}$ levels too low to measure.

Pop received an injection of B$_{12}$ and by the next morning he could sit up by himself. Within two days, he could control his bowels and bladder, and within a week he could play card games and talk coherently on the phone. He didn't make a full recovery—he continued to have a short attention span, and to cry easily—but he didn't need to spend the rest of his life in a nursing home, labeled with "senile dementia."[9]

Unlike Pop, many seniors receive a correct diagnosis for their B$_{12}$-deficiency symptoms only after many months or years of non-diagnosis. That lost time can translate into lost hope; if Pop's doctors had waited even a few more months to detect the cause of his problem, his dementia probably would have been permanent. There appears to be a critical window of opportunity for treating B$_{12}$ deficiency, and therapy started more than six months after the onset of symptoms may fail to reverse these symptoms.

This isn't always true, however, so aggressive treatment is still called for even if symptoms have been present for longer than six months. In one reported case, a patient who'd suffered for nearly a year from "presenile dementia" recovered completely when doctors uncovered and treated his B$_{12}$ deficiency.[10] Also, even at later stages, treatment may prevent additional complications.

Incidentally, while we've put the topic of B$_{12}$-deficiency dementia in our aging chapter, we should note that it can strike even very young people. For instance, doctors reported recently on a twenty-one-year-old woman who developed bipolar disorder and then full-fledged dementia, both due to deficient B$_{12}$ levels and an accompanying folate deficiency. With treatment, her doctors say, she experienced a "dramatic resolution" of her symptoms.[11]

The medical literature even contains reports of infants and toddlers suffering dementia-like symptoms that were reversed, partially or totally, with B$_{12}$ therapy. In these cases, just as with seniors, there is a window of opportunity for effective treatment (see Chapter 6). That's why it's urgent, in either the elderly or the young, to order comprehensive B$_{12}$ testing for any patient exhibiting signs and symptoms of dementia.

Mounting evidence for a B$_{12}$-Alzheimer's link

We differentiate in this chapter between "true" dementias such as Alzheimer's and Pick's, and the often reversible dementia symptoms produced by B$_{12}$ deficiency. Yet preliminary evidence indicates that deficient B$_{12}$ levels worsen Alzheimer's symptoms—and that B$_{12}$ deficiency may even play some role in causing the disease.

Alzheimer's is the most common type of dementia, affecting up to one-fifth of people over eighty and hundreds of thousands of people in their fifties, sixties, and seventies. The diagnosis is confirmed only after patients' deaths, when autopsies reveal the *plaques* (chemical deposits) and *tangles* (malformed nerve cells) that are hallmarks of the disease. While patients are alive, doctors make a tentative diagnosis by excluding other causes of dementia, and using clues provided by brain scans and tests of mental functioning.

Several years ago, Dr. Robert Clarke and colleagues[12] measured the levels of B$_{12}$, folate, and homocysteine in 164 patients diagnosed with Alzheimer's, comparing them to a control group of people without Alzheimer's. (You'll remember that high homocysteine levels are a strong indication of B$_{12}$ deficiency.) At the time the researchers reported their findings, 76 of the 164 patients diagnosed with Alzheimer's had died, and autopsies confirmed the diagnosis; the eighty-eight still-living patients were included as "probable" Alzheimer's cases. Clarke and his colleagues found the following conditions:

- Homocysteine levels at the patients' initial visits were significantly higher in the Alzheimer's group than in control group members.
- B$_{12}$ and folate levels were markedly lower in Alzheimer's patients than in control group members.
- Alzheimer's patients with high homocysteine levels showed greater evidence of disease progression, as revealed by atrophy seen on scans, than those with lower levels. A similar but non-significant trend was seen for serum folate and B$_{12}$ levels.
- Homocysteine levels in the Alzheimer's patients didn't change as the disease progressed, which indicates that the differences between patients and control group members weren't caused by the disease itself, but rather predated or coincided with the onset of Alzheimer's.

Clarke suggests that high levels of toxic homocysteine, possibly stemming from B$_{12}$ deficiency, may cause "microinfarcts"—tiny areas of blood vessel damage—that then trigger the formation of the plaques and tangles that eventually clutter the brain of a person with Alzheimer's. He concludes: "Low blood levels of folate and vitamin B$_{12}$, and elevated total homocysteine (tHcy) levels were associated with Alzheimer's disease. The stability of tHcy levels over time and lack of relationship with duration of symptoms argue against these findings being a consequence of disease and warrant further studies to assess the clinical relevance of these associations for AD."**

More evidence implicating low B$_{12}$ as a player in Alzheimer's comes from a United Kingdom study of a family genetically predisposed to the disease. Remarkably, researchers found that four of six family members with confirmed Alzheimer's had low blood levels of B$_{12}$, while only one of twelve without Alzheimer's exhibited B$_{12}$ deficiency.[13] Another study—this one in Sweden—found that seniors with low intakes of vitamin B$_{12}$ and folate are twice as likely to develop Alzheimer's as people with healthy B$_{12}$ levels. The researchers collected blood samples from their subjects *before* the subjects developed the disease, proving that the low vitamin levels weren't merely a side effect of the Alzheimer's.[14] And one more study, conducted recently in Germany, found that Alzheimer's patients with lower-than-normal B$_{12}$ levels exhibited more behavioral and psychological symptoms of dementia than patients with normal B$_{12}$ levels. "Vitamin B$_{12}$," the researchers concluded, "could play a role in the pathogenesis of behavioral changes in Alzheimer's disease."[15]

An additional clue pointing to a possible link between Alzheimer's and B$_{12}$ comes from Japan, where the normal range for serum B$_{12}$ is set at 500 to 1300 pg/ml—far higher than in the United States. Compared to Americans, the Japanese have a greatly reduced risk of developing Alzheimer's.[16]

If sub-normal B$_{12}$ levels contribute to Alzheimer's, as preliminary evidence suggests, it's crucial that we identify this link quickly. Researchers should pursue the evidence aggressively, and hope that it leads to real progress in treating and/or preventing this insidious disease.

**Unfortunately these researchers did not include MMA testing in their study. The key question that future research must address is: How many patients with confirmed Alzheimer's disease have untreated B$_{12}$ deficiency as evidenced by elevated urinary MMA, the most accurate test?

In the meantime, if you are dealing with a loved one who exhibits symptoms of Alzheimer's, or who suffers from mental deterioration and memory loss in general, your task is simple: *Have the person tested immediately for B$_{12}$ deficiency*. Again, a serum B$_{12}$ test isn't sufficient. Insist on an urinary MMA test as well (see Chapter 10 for a simple explanation of this test). If B$_{12}$ deficiency is causing the symptoms, each day that you wait increases the chances that the damage will become permanent. But even if your loved one is in the late stages of dementia, insist on obtaining accurate B$_{12}$ tests and have the doctor perform a trial of injectable B$_{12,}$ as described in chapters 10 and 11. It won't do any harm, and there's a possibility that it could slow down or halt the progression or even reverse some symptoms. And there's another important reason for the tests: If your relative's dementia turns out to stem from B$_{12}$ deficiency, other family members may be at risk (since B$_{12}$ deficiency often runs in families) and should be tested themselves.

B$_{12}$ deficiency and frequent falls

Dementia is the saddest consequence of undiagnosed B$_{12}$ deficiency, but it's far from the only one. Another is frequent falling, which strips many seniors of their independence and leaves them in wheelchairs or nursing homes.

Falling is the most common cause of fatal injuries among people over sixty-five, with nearly ten thousand seniors dying of fall-related injuries each year. Hospitals treat a third of a million hip fractures every year, most of them in elderly patients, and half of these elderly patients never return home, or live independently, after their injuries.[17]

One reason that B$_{12}$ deficiency is a common cause of falls is that it attacks the nervous system, and particularly the nerves in the lower part of the body. These nerves have an insulating coating known as the myelin sheath, and B$_{12}$ deficiency damages this sheath—in a manner somewhat similar to the fraying of an electrical wire—making it harder for nerve cells to carry messages. As a result, victims often develop weakness, balance problems, leg and back pains, or "glove and stocking" numbness in their hands and feet. Many walk with a slow, foot-slapping gait, because they can't tell when the bottoms of their feet are touching the floor. In addition, B$_{12}$ deficiency can cause dizziness, vertigo, or postural hypotension (a sudden drop in blood pressure upon standing). Together, these problems dramatically increase the risk of falls, and falls in turn can lead to broken bones, hospital stays, and often an end to an independent life.

Arthur came to our emergency department with a nasty gash on his head. He felt weak, he said, and had trouble walking.

It wasn't Arthur's first visit; the seventy-three-year-old's chart showed a history of multiple falls over the past three weeks. After hospitalizing him and running tests to rule out a stroke, the doctors sent Arthur home. He returned five weeks later, again complaining of weakness, and again the doctors discharged him after a short stay.

Nine weeks later, Arthur came in one more time, this time after a fainting episode that led to a serious fall. By this point, his family was considering selling Arthur's home and having him move in with them— an action he dreaded. But this time, an alert doctor ordered a serum B$_{12}$ test, which came back very low, and he started Arthur immediately on B$_{12}$ therapy. Thanks to this doctor's willingness to spend a few extra minutes, Arthur finally obtained a real diagnosis and real help. With B$_{12}$ therapy, it's likely that his weakness will clear up completely, and his chronic falls will become a thing of the past, allowing him to remain independent and keep his home.

Often, as in Arthur's case, older people's falls stem from problems in standing and walking. A typical case, involving a sixty-one-year-old, shows how easy it is to correct these symptoms if they stem from B$_{12}$ deficiency that's detected early enough. This patient first began experiencing numbness and tingling in his toes, which gradually spread throughout his feet. The tingling turned into pain and weakness, and by the time he came to the hospital six months later, he could barely walk with assistance in the daytime, and he couldn't walk at all after dark. (This is a common problem for patients with neurological problems, because when it's dark they can't use their vision to compensate for the impaired sensory input from their feet and legs.)

After quickly identifying this patient's B$_{12}$ deficiency, his new doctors started injections of the vitamin. Within two weeks, the man's tone, strength, and reflexes improved, and within a month, he could walk normally again.[18] In some cases (see Chapter 8), motor problems so severe that they cause near-paralysis can be reversed within a few months.

Such results are common when doctors catch B$_{12}$ deficiency in its early stages. Often, people who could barely walk a few feet are able, within a few months of starting treatment, to resume daily chores, drive, and even exercise again. Equally important, many are able to live independently, without the constant fear of becoming victims of crippling falls that could rob them of their independence.

The benefits to patients are obvious, but there are huge benefits for the medical system and insurers as well. From a financial standpoint, the cost of a fall and resulting fracture—emergency department visit, X rays, labs, CT scans, casting, admission, possible surgery, physical therapy, medications, a visiting nurse, and possible placement in an extended care facility—far exceeds the cost of blood or urine tests to ascertain if vitamin B_{12} deficiency exists. In 2003, the cost of a hip fracture was approximately $54,000 (see Appendix V).

We find it perplexing that hospitals do not routinely provide B_{12} screening for patients with weakness or repeated falls, particularly in light of the fact that the diagnostic procedures that hospitals *do* order for these patients are so expensive. For example, patients with these symptoms almost always receive a CT scan of the brain, costing approximately $1,000, and each time they return, they receive additional scans. We have no quarrel with ordering expensive CT scans, which can reveal problems other than B_{12} deficiency (although they're useless for diagnosing low B_{12}); rather, we have a problem with medical professionals who fail to order equally necessary and far less expensive B_{12} tests.

Arthur, for example, had $3,000 worth of CT scans in five months, and his total hospital bill exceeded $30,000, when less than $100 for a urinary MMA test on his first visit would have identified his B_{12} deficiency. If he'd suffered a fracture, the three-day hospital stay for his surgery in 1999 would have cost more than $14,000, not including the surgeon's bill or post hospital rehabilitation.

Of course, not all falls stem from B_{12} deficiency, but statistics suggest that a significant percentage do. Thus, doctors should test for this disorder any time an older patient complains of pain, numbness, weakness, dizziness, difficulty in walking, or falls.

The B_{12}–osteoporosis connection

In 2004, newspapers and national newscasts showcased three new studies showing a strong link between low B_{12} levels and osteoporosis, one of the leading cripplers of seniors. Osteoporosis causes a thinning and weakening of the bones, often leading to debilitating or even fatal fractures.

The first study, which evaluated hip-bone mineral density in eighty-three elderly women, found that those with the lowest levels of B_{12} exhibited much more rapid hip bone loss than those with higher B_{12} levels. Lead author Dr. Katie Stone commented, "We knew that vitamin B_{12} benefited the nervous system, but our findings suggest that it may also benefit bone health."[19]

The two other studies both reported a strong association between high homocysteine levels and bone fractures. (As we've explained, one of the primary causes of high homocysteine is low B_{12}.) One study following nearly 2,000 men and women for two decades found that men with the highest concentrations of homocysteine were nearly four times as likely to break a hip as were those with the lowest concentrations, while the risk for women with the highest homocysteine levels was double that of women with the lowest levels. The researchers reporting this finding noted, "If the homocysteine concentration truly is a causal mechanism for the risk of fracture, the public health implications could be substantial."[20]

The other study, involving more than 2,400 Dutch subjects, found that men and women with the highest homocysteine concentrations were twice as likely to break a hip, or experience other commonly broken bones as were those with lower homocysteine.[21]

While these new studies were treated as ground-breaking, previous research had already established a powerful connection between B_{12} deficiency and osteoporosis. It's well documented that people with untreated pernicious anemia are at high risk for osteoporosis and resulting fractures,[22] which is not surprising because vitamin B_{12} is crucial to the function of osteoblasts (bone-forming cells). In one case study, a patient with severe osteoporosis exhibited a "dramatic response" to treatment with B_{12} and cyclic etidronate (a bone-strengthening drug), with serial bone density measurements demonstrating a 15 percent and 17 percent increase in the lumbar (lower back) and greater trochanter (hip) regions, respectively, and a 79 percent increase in the femoral neck region, over the two-year follow-up period—an effect significantly greater than that which would be expected with etidronate alone. In addition, the patient suffered no new fractures during the course of the study.[23]

Given all of these findings, it is our opinion that tests for B_{12} deficiency should be a standard part of the evaluation for any patient with osteoporosis—and in particular for patients who are at high risk of falls, or who have already suffered falls and/or sustained fractures. Moreover, research on the connection between low B$_{12}$ and increased risk for fall-related injuries, fractures, and osteoporosis needs to become a national priority. The evidence indicates that B$_{12}$ deficiency is epidemic among seniors; that low B$_{12}$ and high homocysteine are strong risk factors for osteoporosis; that B$_{12}$ deficiency also leads to falls and injuries by impairing neurological function; and that B$_{12}$ therapy may help stop or reverse bone loss, and can often reverse neurological dysfunction, in B$_{12}$-deficient patients. Translating these research findings into a national effort to combat B$_{12}$ deficiency in seniors could lead to a significant drop in the numbers of crippling or fatal falls suffered by the elderly—and an equally large drop in America's health-care costs.

Other B$_{12}$ ills that masquerade as aging

In Chapter 5, we'll further discuss how low B$_{12}$ levels increase levels of homocysteine, and how high levels of this toxic amino acid can harm the heart, circulatory system, and immune system. This can contribute to congestive heart failure, coronary artery disease, transient ischemic attacks (TIAs or "mini-strokes"), cerebral vascular accidents (strokes), heart attacks, and deep vein thromboses—all problems that plague the elderly, in particular.

But B$_{12}$ deficiency disables its older victims in still more ways. The nervous system impairment stemming from this deficiency can cause tremors, handwriting difficulties, and other symptoms severe enough to resemble the early stages of Parkinson's disease. (See Chapter 3 for more on this.) And, because B$_{12}$ deficiency affects all of the nerves, it can also affect the nerves of the eye and lead to reduced vision or even blindness. In young adults, blindness caused by B$_{12}$ deficiency is so unexpected that it often leads to an accurate diagnosis. But the elderly, and especially diabetics, aren't as lucky: If their failing eyesight stems from B$_{12}$ deficiency, it's likely to be attributed to age or diabetic eye damage. New research, while preliminary, also links B$_{12}$ deficiency to one form of cataracts.[24]

Again, these disorders have many causes, and B$_{12}$ deficiency is just one of them. But even if only one in seven seniors suffers from problems linked to deficient B$_{12}$ levels—and that's likely to be a substantial underestimate—identifying and treating these individuals can save billions of dollars, and, more important, improve or even save millions of lives. The moral for medical professionals is clear: We owe it to our patients to diagnose B_{12} deficiency, and save our patients from preventable debility or death.

Notes

1. Schmidt, cited in "Americans lack critical knowledge about potentially debilitating condition," *Doctor's Guide,* November 19, 1997 (http://www.docguide.com), .
2. Carmel, R. Prevalence of undiagnosed pernicious anemia in the elderly. *Archives of Internal Medicine* 1996, 156(10):1097–1100.
3. Norman, E.J. and Morrison, J.A. Incidence estimate of cobalamin deficiency in independently living elderly subjects using the urinary methylmalonic acid assay. *Blood* 1993, 82(10 Suppl 1):1850.
4. Norman, Eric. Vitamin B_{12} deficiency. *Journal of Family Practice* (1993), 36:597.
5. Walker III, Sydney. *Dose of Sanity*. New York: John Wiley & Sons, 1996, p. 192.
6. Lopponen, M., Raiha, I., Isoaho, R., Vahlberg, T., and Kivela, S. L. Diagnosing cognitive impairment and dementia in primary health care—a more active approach is needed. *Age and Ageing*, 32(6):606–12.
7. Interview with Mark Goodman in *Clinical Pearls News* (1997), 7(10):132-134.
8. Teunisse, S., Bollen, A. E., Van Gool, W. A., Walstra, G. J. M. Dementia and subnormal levels of vitamin B_{12}: effects of replacement therapy on dementia. *Journal of Neurology* (1996), 243(7):522–529.
9. Bernstein, Leslie. Vital signs: Dementia without a cause. *Discover* (February 2000), 21(2):31–2.
10. Cited by Hector, Melvin, and Burton, John, What are the psychiatric manifestations of vitamin B_{12} deficiency? *Journal of the American Geriatrics Society* (1988), 36:1105–1112.
11. Reid, S. D. Pseudodementia in a twenty-one-year-old with bipolar disorder and vitamin B_{12} and folate deficiency. *West Indian Medical Journal* (2000), 49(4):347–8.
12. Clarke, R., Smith, A. D., Jobst, K. A., Refsum, H., Sutton, L., and Ueland, P. M. Folate, vitamin B_{12} and serum total homocysteine levels in confirmed Alzheimer's disease. *Archives of Neurology* (1998), 55:1449–55.
13. McCaddon, A., and Kelly, C. L. Familial Alzheimer's disease and vitamin B_{12} deficiency. *Age and Ageing* (1994), 23(4):334–7.
14. Wang, H-X., Wahlin, A., Basun, H., Fastbom, J., Winblad, B., and Fratiglioni, L. Vitamin B_{12} and folate in relation to the development of Alzheimer's disease. *Neurology* 2001, 56:1188–94.
15. Meins, W., Muller-Thomsen, T., and Meier-Baumgartnerm, H. P. Subnormal serum vitamin B_{12} and behavioural and psychological symptoms in

Alzheimer's disease. *International Journal of Geriatric Psychiatry* (2000), 15(5):415– 8.

16. Dommisse, J. V. Vitamin B$_{12}$. *Primary Psychiatry* 1996, 3(4):18–21.

17. Statistics are from "Falls and hip fractures among older adults," Centers for Disease Control and Prevention, November 2000, http://www.cdc.gov.

18. Karantanas, A. H., Markonis, A., and Bisbiyiannis, G. Subacute combined degeneration of the spinal cord with involvement of the anterior columns: A new MRI finding. *Neuroradiology* (2000), 42:115–117.

19. Stone, K. L., Bauer, D. C., Sellmeyer, D., and Cummings, S. R. Low serum vitamin B$_{12}$ levels are associated with increased hip bone loss in older women: A prospective study. *Journal of Clinical Endocrinology & Metabolism* 2004, 89(3): 1217–21.

20. McLean, R. R., et al. Homocysteine as a predictive factor for hip fracture in older persons. *New England Journal of Medicine* 2004, 350:2042–2049.

21. van Meurs, J. B. J., et al. Homocysteine levels and the risk of osteoporotic fracture. *New England Journal of Medicine* 2004, 350:2033–41.

22. Goerss, J. B., et al. Risk of fractures in patients with pernicious anemia. *J Bone Miner Res* 1992 May; 7(5):573–9. Espallargues, M., et al. Identifying bone-mass related risk factors for fracture to guide bone densitometry measurements: A systematic review of the literature. *Osteoporosis Int.* 2001;12(10):811–22.

23. Mellton, M. E., and Kochman, M. L. Reversal of severe osteoporosis with vitamin B12 and etidronate therapy in a patient with pernicious anemia. *Metabolism* 1995, 43(4):468–9.

24. Kuzniarz, M., Mitchell, P., Cumming, R. G., and Flood, V. M. Use of vitamin supplements and cataract: The Blue Mountains Eye Study. *American Journal of Ophthalmology* (2001), 132:19–26.

Deadly Mimic: When B_{12} Deficiency Masquerades as Multiple Sclerosis or Other Neurological Disorders

"...Eighty to 90 percent of untreated patients [suffering from a deficiency of vitamin B_{12}] will develop disorders of the nervous system."
—E. Steve Roach, M.D., and William T. McLean, M.D.[1]

B_{12} deficiency strikes large numbers of seniors, but if you think that it's solely an "old person's disease," think again. A deficiency of B_{12} can destroy your nervous system at any age, and we've seen children, teens, young adults, and middle-aged people crippled or killed by this preventable disease.

Neurologic symptoms of B_{12} deficiency in young adults (or in children, see Chapter 6) often baffle doctors, particularly when blood tests are normal and symptoms are subtle. The result, frequently, is a dangerous delay in obtaining treatment. But even if you show obvious signs and symptoms of B_{12} deficiency, there's no guarantee that you'll get a quick diagnosis.

After he'd spent years suffering from odd and frightening symptoms that a neurologist finally diagnosed, Washington Post *writer Thomas Heath described "how close my bewildering illness had come to killing me." [2]*

Barely into his forties, and seemingly in excellent health, Heath began experiencing memory lapses and numbness in his hands and lower legs. His thinking deteriorated to the point that his wife suspected early-onset

Alzheimer's. He started losing his balance, and stopped running because he kept falling. Later, he began losing control of his bowels and bladder.

When a physical showed that Heath had low folic acid levels, one doctor put him on folate supplements—which can mask B$_{12}$ deficiency. Another physician attributed his painful tongue, a classic sign of B$_{12}$ deficiency, to a fungus infection. When walking became difficult, Heath went to an orthopedic doctor who gave him steroids, which can also mask B$_{12}$ deficiency. A psychiatrist spent several hours trying to coax him into taking antidepressant medications.

Finally, after more than three years of non-diagnosis, Heath went to a neurologist. By then, he was a wreck. "When he asked me to close my eyes and walk a straight line, I almost fell over," Heath says. "I couldn't tell where my legs were without my sight." The doctor, eventually suspecting B$_{12}$ deficiency, sent Health to a hematologist who quickly said two words that saved Heath's life: "pernicious anemia."

Heath immediately started B$_{12}$ injections, and his hands are now completely functional. He can jog again, but only slowly. (He ran marathons before he became ill.) He enjoys books and movies now, but says, "I still seem to have more trouble than usual remembering names, words and appointments." Despite his continuing debility, Heath says he's fortunate: "Although my body, my life, and my marriage were slowly unraveling because of this insidious disease, they have been repaired."

Heath's diagnosis came far later than it should have, but he is luckier than others who never get diagnosed, and who suffer or even die without ever knowing that their problems were curable. Physician Robert Schilling cites the tragic case of a thirty-five-year-old man doomed to spend the rest of his life on a Stryker frame (a rotating bed for patients who cannot move) because "no one had thought of vitamin B$_{12}$ deficiency until it was too late."[3] And Heath is lucky that he suffered from "classic" pernicious anemia, rather than other, subtler forms of B$_{12}$ deficiency that doctors (including neurologists) often misdiagnose.

Such misdiagnoses occur for several reasons. One is that the symptoms of B$_{12}$ deficiency are easy to mistake for symptoms of other neurologic diseases, such as amyotrophic lateral sclerosis (ALS, also known as Lou Gehrig's disease) or multiple sclerosis (see next section). Another is that, as we've noted, doctors typically look for blood abnormalities when they check for B$_{12}$ deficiency—but *neurological damage can precede blood anomalies by years or even decades*. Still another reason for missed diagnoses is that even doctors somewhat knowledgeable about B$_{12}$ deficiency think of it as a rare disease, or a disease of old age. Those doctors, however, are wrong, because B$_{12}$ deficiency is common, has many causes, and strikes people of all ages.

Because B$_{12}$ deficiency mimics so many other disorders, doctors can't rule out a deficiency simply by examining patients. With the right tests, however, an informed and conscientious doctor can make the right call in a matter of days—and that diagnosis can lead to a dramatic cure. In one case, for instance, mystified doctors sent a twenty-eight-year-old woman to physician Helmut Wilhelm after she developed unexplained vision loss. In addition to checking the woman for other common causes of sudden blindness, Wilhelm discovered that her serum B$_{12}$ levels were only one-third of the normal limit. He started vitamin B$_{12}$ injections immediately, leading to "an almost complete recovery."[4]

If You Suffer from these Symptoms... Could It Be B$_{12}$ Deficiency?

The neurological symptoms of B$_{12}$ deficiency that occur in young and middle-aged people are very similar to those in older people. They include the following:

• Tremor, often misdiagnosed as essential tremor or pre-Parkinson's disease

• Paralysis, sometimes attributed to Guillain-Barré syndrome

• Pain, fatigue, and debility, often labeled as "chronic fatigue syndrome"

• "Shaky leg" syndrome (leg trembling)

• Confusion and mental fogginess, often misdiagnosed as early-onset dementia

• Unsteadiness, dizziness, numbness and tingling, often misdiagnosed as multiple sclerosis

• Psychiatric symptoms, such as depression or psychosis (covered in greater length in the next chapter)

• Vision loss or blindness

In contrast, a doctor ignorant about the effects of B$_{12}$ deficiency can destroy a patient's life. John Hotchkiss, Jr., M.D., a crusader for the accurate diagnosis of B$_{12}$-deficient patients, offers an example. When Hotchkiss (an ear-nose-throat specialist, now retired) practiced in a medical group, one of his partners—a Harvard graduate—objected strenuously to Hotchkiss's insistence on ruling out B$_{12}$ deficiency in patients with neurological disorders or other suspicious signs and symptoms. The doctor grew hostile on more than one occasion when Hotchkiss suggested evaluating a patient's B$_{12}$ levels, and he refused to be swayed by the medical literature Hotchkiss sent him.

"Some years later," Hotchkiss says, "he sent a patient to me for 'dizziness' evaluation." Hotchkiss discovered that the woman was not dizzy, but instead suffered from poor coordination stemming from neurological dysfunction. He wasn't surprised; the woman's history included a gastrectomy twelve years earlier, a surgery that inevitably results in severe B$_{12}$ deficiency if patients don't receive compensatory B$_{12}$ injections.

The woman had been followed by Hotchkiss's colleague ever since the surgery, Hotchkiss says, "but he had done no follow-up studies concerning her B$_{12}$ status." As a result, she suffered from a condition known as "combined systems disease" or "subacute combined degeneration," a complication of chronic B$_{12}$ deficiency in which damage to the spinal cord tracts causes irreversible crippling.

"The doctor not only failed to monitor her and prevent this from happening, a grave dereliction, but he failed to recognize the condition when it occurred," Hotchkiss says. "When we met in the hall some weeks later, he said, 'You got me.'"[5]

Hotchkiss's story is further evidence that even specialists can miss a simple diagnosis of B$_{12}$ deficiency. It also demonstrates that even the most prestigious doctors, trained at the best schools, aren't immune from this failing. In addition, it's an illustration of why early treatment is crucial. This patient, of course, never should have developed symptoms to begin with, but once she did, a quick diagnosis would have saved her health.

Erica, a personal friend of ours, developed a mild tremor and arm weakness in middle age. When two neurologists failed to diagnose her problem, her son, a physician himself, stepped in and ordered tests that *identified a B_{12} deficiency. He immediately began treatment, and four years later, her tremor is reduced by more than 75 percent and her arm no longer feels weak. The damage done by her B_{12} deficiency was at least partially reversible, and even more important, it will never progress to the point where she will suffer dementia, paralysis, or other crippling symptoms.*

If you suffer from neurological symptoms, the only way to rule out B_{12} deficiency is by insisting that a doctor—whether it's your family practitioner, neurologist, psychiatrist, or other specialist—order a urinary MMA, a serum B_{12}, and a homocysteine test to accurately determine your B_{12} status. The alternative—never knowing if your symptoms could stem from a diagnosable, treatable, and often fully curable disorder—is simply unacceptable.

Is it multiple sclerosis or B_{12} deficiency?

Kathy* was just twenty-one when she fractured her leg. It healed, but afterward, it felt numb and Kathy found it harder and harder to walk. Then her fingers began tingling, and she started dropping objects frequently. Soon her right foot began dragging when she walked.

A doctor checked Kathy's serum B_{12} level, which was "normal," although she was anemic and her red blood cells were large, a sign of B_{12} deficiency. Her bone marrow appeared normal, and a repeat B_{12} test also came back "normal." Reviewing these findings, Kathy's doctor told her the bad news: She had multiple sclerosis (MS), a tragic diagnosis for a young woman. Barely out of her teens, Kathy faced a life burdened by a crippling disease that might eventually leave her paralyzed.

Six years later, however, Kathy found out her doctor was wrong.

When Kathy turned twenty-seven, a new bone marrow test showed abnormalities consistent with B_{12} deficiency. Her iron deficiency anemia was growing worse, and her red blood cells were still enlarged. A new doctor reviewed Kathy's history from birth, spotting her early delays in walking and reading, and her poor coordination—as well as her mother's two unsuccessful pregnancies (one ending in a miscarriage, and the other in a stillbirth), and her father's history of hyperthyroidism and early death from heart disease. In his mind, Kathy's current symptoms

---

*Our pseudonym for the patient cited in this journal report.

and past history added up not to multiple sclerosis but to a familial form of B₁₂ deficiency. Further tests indeed showed that she suffered from a hereditary defect of B₁₂ metabolism, called cobalamin G, a diagnosis her previous doctors had missed for twenty-seven years.

Kathy's doctor started her on weekly B₁₂ shots, and gave her another medication (oral betaine) to normalize the high homocysteine levels caused by her inborn error of B₁₂ metabolism. Her weakness lessened, and after time she began walking more easily. But according to the physician who reported her case in the New England Journal of Medicine, *she continued to suffer from permanent neurologic damage—a legacy of more than a quarter-century of misdiagnosis.[6]*

Your coffee pot and your vacuum cleaner run on electricity, carried through wires. A thin layer of insulation covers these wires, preventing the current from escaping to the outside and disrupting the flow of electricity.

Similarly, the neurons in your brain and spinal cord send electrical messages. They too are insulated, by a protective fatty coating called *myelin*. If this myelin breaks down, or becomes swollen, the electrical impulses sent by neurons can go haywire. One common cause of this short-circuiting is multiple sclerosis (MS), a disease that most often strikes young or middle-aged people, most of them women and most of them Caucasian.

We don't know what causes multiple sclerosis. We know that it's an autoimmune disease, possibly triggered by exposure to a virus, in which the body mistakenly attacks its own cells. We know that genes play a role, because having a first-degree relative with MS increases the risk of developing the disease several-fold. And we know that geography is involved: People born above the 40th parallel in the northern hemisphere, or below the 40th parallel in the southern hemisphere, have a higher risk of developing MS than people near the equator, unless they move before puberty.

We know, too, that multiple sclerosis and B₁₂ deficiency are different disorders. But the conditions are linked in three crucial ways:

- The symptoms of B₁₂ deficiency sometimes mimic the symptoms of multiple sclerosis, leading to misdiagnosis—a mistake with grave consequences, because B₁₂ deficiency is completely reversible in its early stages, while MS is incurable.

- MS and chronic untreated B$_{12}$ deficiency both damage myelin, causing lesions or disease in the brain and spinal cord.
- Scientists report intriguing evidence tentatively implicating low B$_{12}$ levels in the development or exacerbation of multiple sclerosis—meaning that even when MS is diagnosed correctly, B$_{12}$ deficiency could possibly be contributing to the disease.

Later, we'll outline the speculative evidence implicating deficient B$_{12}$ levels as a factor in true cases of multiple sclerosis. First, however, let's look at why some of the 300,000 Americans diagnosed with MS may, instead, be suffering from a B$_{12}$ deficiency that can be diagnosed and cured.

Is it MS or B$_{12}$ deficiency?

Diagnosing multiple sclerosis is a challenge because no test can prove or rule out the presence of the disease, and because many other disorders mimic its signs and symptoms. It's estimated, in fact, that as many as ten percent of people diagnosed with multiple sclerosis *don't actually have the disease.*[7]

Of this group—which translates into as many as 30,000 Americans—a significant number are likely to have B$_{12}$ deficiency. The resemblance between MS and B$_{12}$ deficiency is striking, with common symptoms including the following:

- gait problems
- numbness
- "pins and needles" sensations
- depression, paranoia, or psychosis
- memory loss, and other cognitive changes
- weight loss
- tremors
- fatigue
- coordination problems
- incontinence
- pain
- vision loss

As we noted, there's a simple reason for this resemblance. Multiple sclerosis stems from myelin damage—and B$_{12}$ deficiency, left untreated long enough, also damages myelin, causing the same "short-circuiting" of nerve impulses.

But here's the big difference: When myelin destruction stems from B$_{12}$ deficiency, we can cure the patient's symptoms—all of them—if we catch the problem in time. Thus, it stands to reason that doctors should always rule out B$_{12}$ deficiency in patients with MS. Yet current standards of care do *not* dictate that doctors order the tests needed to do this, and many, as a result, never do.

Accurate diagnosis requires ordering a battery of tests that can conclusively prove, or definitively rule out, B$_{12}$ deficiency (see list at the end of this chapter). Even a "definitive" diagnosis of MS based on abnormal MRI findings does not eliminate the need for testing. As physician Robert Schilling notes, "Even though magnetic resonance imaging has been a significant advance in the diagnosis of multiple sclerosis, the findings are not 100 percent specific and cannot be relied on to differentiate MS from cobalamin [B$_{12}$] deficiency or another condition."[8]

Unfortunately, most doctors "rule out" B$_{12}$ deficiency in patients with suspected MS simply by ordering a serum B$_{12}$ test, which can be grossly inaccurate. (Remember that this test can show normal or even high B$_{12}$ levels in markedly deficient patients.) Worse yet, many fail to order any tests at all to rule out B$_{12}$ deficiency.

The results can be catastrophic, and for the seventy-seven-year-old woman we first mentioned in Chapter 2, they're likely to be fatal. Doctors told this woman when she was in her late fifties that she had MS, even though the disease typically strikes people below the age of fifty. One doctor gave her monthly B$_{12}$ shots for years—during which time her symptoms stabilized—but a new doctor discontinued them around the time of her seventy-second birthday. She deteriorated drastically over the next five years, finally arriving in the emergency room suffering from dementia and respiratory failure. Tests revealed clear evidence of B$_{12}$ deficiency, including an elevated MMA, anemia, and hypersegmented neutrophils, but by then it was too late to save her. When we saw her, she was comatose and rolled into a fetal position. She had large bedsores and a severe blood infection (sepsis). She will spend the remainder of her life in an institution under hospice care.

Sadly, this woman's case is not an isolated anomaly. Robert Schilling and William Williams wrote in 1995, "Many experienced hematologists have seen patients with severe, permanent neurologic damage because the B$_{12}$ deficiency was mistaken for another disorder, such as *multiple sclerosis* [italics added], diabetic neuropathy, amyotrophic lateral sclerosis, or even Guillain-Barré syndrome." One of Schilling's own cases involved a woman diagnosed with MS eight months earlier by another doctor. The tests ordered by Schilling revealed conclusively that the woman suffered from a B$_{12}$ deficiency, and did not have multiple sclerosis.[9]

Similarly, Dr. Eric Norman reported in 2000 that of six young women his research team diagnosed with B$_{12}$ deficiency, three were initially suspected of having MS. These three women's original doctors were puzzled and diagnosis was delayed because of the similarities between MS and B$_{12}$ deficiency, and because their patients were young. Norman comments, "This population deserves further evaluations since it has not been considered prone to cobalamin [B$_{12}$] deficiency." Correct treatment of these six patients resulted in a nearly complete recovery for two women, and partial recovery in one other case. The extent of improvement in two other women could not be measured since treatment had just begun when the report was published, and the last woman had not yet developed significant neurologic symptoms.[10]

How many similar cases of B$_{12}$ deficiency are misdiagnosed as MS? We don't know, but cases reported in the medical literature make it clear that the problem isn't an isolated one.

In the American Journal of Psychiatry[11] *Gary Payinda and colleagues reported the case of a woman who probably owes them her life—and certainly owes them her sanity.*

At fifty-two years of age, Mrs. A suddenly developed paralysis in her legs. Her doctor referred her to a neurologist, who diagnosed her with multiple sclerosis. Over the next two months, Mrs. A was placed on numerous medications, but her leg weakness progressed and the drugs did not help. She required a cane, then used a walker, and eventually needed a wheelchair to get around. As time went by, Mrs. A became agitated and angry. She grew paranoid, and she called the police to report that her family was trying to poison her. She also became violent, throwing furniture and even trying to jump from a moving car.

Mrs. A's family, stunned and frightened by her worsening behavior, finally took her to an emergency psychiatric center. She appeared di-

sheveled, was delirious and disoriented, and paranoid, and could not stand without assistance. The psychiatric facility obtained a B$_{12}$ level, which came back extremely low *at 9pg/ml (normal is 200-950).*

The doctors diagnosed Mrs. A. with subacute combined spinal cord degeneration and psychosis due to a severe vitamin B$_{12}$ deficiency. Additional tests revealed that she suffered from pernicious anemia; earlier physicians missed the diagnosis in part because her folic acid supplements had masked her blood abnormalities.

Two days after starting B$_{12}$ injections, Mrs. A started regaining the strength in her legs. Within eight weeks, her symptoms of mental illness vanished. Unfortunately, she may never fully regain her health and mobility, because of the delay in diagnosing her correctly. The cause of that delay: her original neurologist failed to diagnose her correctly, instead misdiagnosing her with MS and apparently never considering B$_{12}$ deficiency.

Patients like Mrs. A suffer terribly, and unnecessarily, because many physicians lack even the most basic knowledge about B$_{12}$-deficiency symptoms. Moreover, this ignorance isn't limited to inexperienced doctors. Recently, we found a noted neurologist offering the following advice to fellow doctors on differentiating between MS and B$_{12}$ deficiency:

"Multiple sclerosis often has the pattern of relapse then [remission] with multiple episodes. B$_{12}$ deficiency progressively worsens.... Multiple sclerosis can have other systems affected—for example, visual, coordination, tremor—and often years apart from the current problem. These are not features of B$_{12}$ deficiency.... In most cases history and exam can tell these two apart, but sometimes one can mimic the other. If so, part of the workup could include a B$_{12}$ level and if suspicion is high, one can check homocysteine and methylmalonic acid levels, metabolites which are more sensitive for B$_{12}$ deficiency—these tests should give an answer if any question of B$_{12}$ deficiency exists."[12]

What's wrong with this advice, offered by a physician at a leading American hospital? Almost everything. Here's why:

- B$_{12}$ deficiency can easily mimic the remission-and-relapse pattern of MS. A patient getting blood transfusions, or receiving tube or IV feedings, can receive enough B$_{12}$ to temporarily replenish B$_{12}$ levels. A B$_{12}$-deficient vegetarian who starts eating more animal products or meat again can appear to go into "remission." Steroids administered to patients during an "attack" can increase B$_{12}$ absorption in undiagnosed autoimmune pernicious anemia patients, again mimicking remission.** A patient who starts taking high-dose vitamins may receive enough B$_{12}$ to cause improvement. Doctors who give occasional B$_{12}$ injections, "just in case you need it," can make patients' symptoms vanish temporarily, only to return when the shots' effects wear off. Conversely, stress, pregnancy, infection, administration of immunizations with mercury (see Chapter 12), exposure to nitrous oxide, or a switch to a vegetarian diet can cause a "relapse." Thus, arbitrarily ruling out B$_{12}$ deficiency in a patient with a relapsing and remitting pattern of MS symptoms can be deadly.

• A history and exam are *never* sufficient to rule out B$_{12}$ deficiency in a patient with suspected MS, because B$_{12}$ deficiency can mimic the signs and symptoms of even classic MS.

• Vision problems (up to and including blindness), tremor, and poor coordination can indeed be symptoms of B$_{12}$ deficiency, and the pattern and timing of symptoms can vary from patient to patient—just as in multiple sclerosis.

• Suggesting that the workup for a patient with multiple sclerosis "*could include* a B$_{12}$ level [italics added]," as though the test is optional, is dangerously misguided. This test, and a urinary MMA and Hcy, are all absolute necessities in every suspected case of MS.

• The recommendation that only patients whose MS diagnosis is obviously "suspicious" should receive MMA and homocysteine tests is, again, potentially deadly. As we've explained, the standard serum B$_{12}$ test is often inaccurate. Moreover, tests

---

**G. R. Lee states in *Wintrobe's Clinical Hematology* (1999, 10th Edition, pp. 941–958), "The fact that some patients with pernicious anemia respond to the administration of adrenal corticosteroids also suggests a possible autoimmune mechanism in the development of the disease. The reported responses include hematologic improvement, increased vitamin B$_{12}$ absorption, histologic improvement in gastric mucosa, appearance of acid and intrinsic factor in gastric juice and decrease in serum titers of intrinsic factor antibody."

for anemia and enlarged red blood cells can be misleading because—and this is a critical piece of information that most doctors lack—the steroids commonly used to treat multiple sclerosis can normalize the anemia and enlarged cells characteristic of B$_{12}$, while allowing the neurologic damage to continue unchecked. (This is similar to the effects of folic acid supplementation, which we discussed earlier.)

Thus, in our opinion, a doctor must rule out B$_{12}$ deficiency in all patients suspected of having MS, or actually diagnosed with MS, by ordering tests for urinary MMA, Hcy, and serum B$_{12}$ levels. Failing to order these tests puts patients at risk for permanent injury or even death, and in our opinion constitutes negligence.

As medical professionals, we've seen the results of this negligence firsthand. One case involved Linda, a thirty-six-year-old patient diagnosed with MS. Linda turned up in the emergency room three years after her initial diagnosis (and several months after delivering a baby), when her symptoms began growing worse. She complained of foggy vision and weakness in her legs, and she'd fallen and injured her left knee.

The tests the ER doctor ordered for Linda revealed a very low B$_{12}$ level. It's likely that Linda's B$_{12}$ stores became dangerously depleted during her pregnancy, triggering the exacerbation of her symptoms. But when the ER doctor notified Linda's neurologist that her B$_{12}$ level was very low, and could be causing some or all of her symptoms, the neurologist replied brusquely, "No, this patient has documented MS."

In an age of managed-care cost cutting, many physicians consider comprehensive testing for B$_{12}$ deficiency "too expensive," although in reality the cost of *not* performing these tests is vastly higher. Copaxone, a drug for MS that must be injected daily, costs approximately $15,000 per year; Betaseron and Avonex are nearly as expensive, at $14,000 and $12,000 per year, respectively. In addition, many people with MS require extensive and expensive therapy, and some require long-term care. If even a small percentage of cases diagnosed as MS involve B$_{12}$ deficiency, correct diagnosis could save families, and the American medical system, millions of dollars annually.

When it comes to B$_{12}$ screening, however, physicians and managed care providers are often penny-wise and pound-foolish. Thus, if you've been diagnosed with multiple sclerosis, or if a doctor suggests that your symptoms point to MS, it's up to you to be assertive and insist on thor-

The Cost of Misdiagnosis

Three hundred thousand Americans currently are diagnosed with multiple sclerosis. If only 4.2 percent of them actually suffer from B$_{12}$ deficiency—the lowest estimate we can find in the medical literature, and undoubtedly a gross underestimate because no urinary MMAs were performed and the researcher used outdated homocysteine cutoff scores too high to diagnose many other cases[13]—that adds up to 12,600 people.

Using this lowest-possible estimate, let's look at the cost of treating these individuals:

• If these 12,600 people take Betaseron, at $14,000 per year, the cost is: 176 million dollars yearly.
• If these 12,600 people eventually require nursing home care, the cost is: 630 million dollars yearly.
• If these 12,600 people receive a correct diagnosis, the cost of their treatment (including fifty-dollar office visits to receive monthly B$_{12}$ injections, plus the cost of the injections) drops to: less than eight million dollars yearly.
• And, if these 12,600 people administer the shots themselves (just as most of them now inject their own MS drugs), the cost drops to: $302,000 yearly!

ough testing. Don't assume that your doctor will check you for B$_{12}$ deficiency, and don't assume—even if your doctor says you'll be tested—that he or she will order the right tests. Instead, obtain your test results, check them against the list at the end of this chapter, and keep pushing until every test on the list is performed. Don't take the risk of being diagnosed with an incurable disease, when you may have one that's completely curable in its early stages.

George, a fifty-two-year-old male, came into the ER with an injured right foot. Wheelchair-bound due to symptoms of MS, George could get up to shave and go to the bathroom, and that's what he'd been doing when he fell and broke his foot. His legs were very weak, and he walked with a spastic gait when he moved from his wheelchair to a regular chair. He complained of chronic mid-back pain and told the ER staff that in addition to his MS (diagnosed eighteen months earlier), he suffered from depression, bipolar disorder, spinal stenosis, an irritable bowel, and neuralgia.

George's history raised red flags, leading the ER doctor to look for additional evidence of B$_{12}$ deficiency. George's blood tests showed enlarged red blood cells, and his MMA came back elevated. The latter clearly indicated B$_{12}$ deficiency, particularly after the doctor ruled out other likely causes of high serum MMA, such as impaired kidney function. Interestingly, George had high serum B$_{12}$ levels, possibly because other doctors—mistaking his symptoms for effects of alcoholism—occasionally gave him intravenous fluids containing vitamins.

The ER doctor called George's primary care doctor one week later, after receiving all of George's results, and explained that the findings indicated that B$_{12}$ deficiency was causing or exacerbating George's symptoms. George's doctor was grateful for the information, saying, "I owe you one."

Speculation: Does true MS involve a B$_{12}$ abnormality?

MS and B$_{12}$ deficiency are two different diseases, and doctors diagnose the great majority of cases of MS correctly. Yet intriguing (although highly speculative) clues are now leading scientists to explore the possibility that even classic multiple sclerosis may involve a defect in B$_{12}$ metabolism.

Interestingly, there are many similarities between MS and pernicious anemia, the autoimmune form of B$_{12}$ deficiency we described in Chapter 1. The two diseases strike both young adults*** and middle-aged persons, and both involve immune system abnormalities. Both are more common in cold northern areas than in tropical southern areas, and both affect Caucasians more often than African Americans. Both diseases strike females more often than males, and in the same ratio (1.3 to 1). There are more links, too, between multiple sclerosis and B$_{12}$ deficiency:

• Enlarged red blood cells, a classic sign of B$_{12}$ deficiency,

---

***Although it is not well known or extensively documented, autoimmune pernicious anemia can strike people in their twenties, thirties, and forties. Because physicians believe that pernicious anemia typically strikes in the fifth or sixth decade of life, they rarely evaluate young adults for this disease, instead assuming that the neurological symptoms of B$_{12}$ deficiency or pernicious anemia are caused by multiple sclerosis.

often occur in MS patients. This abnormal finding is seen even in the earliest stages of MS, and thus isn't likely to be merely a side effect of the disease.

• Researchers often report marginal serum levels of B$_{12}$ in MS patients.

• B$_{12}$ injections do not improve motor function in most people with true MS. However, one study of MS patients found that visual and brain stem auditory evoked potentials—measurements of the nervous system's response to stimuli—improved more frequently during B$_{12}$ treatment than before treatment.[14] (Unfortunately, it's impossible to know if the motor symptoms of the patients in this study might also have improved if B$_{12}$ treatment had been started earlier, before their myelin damage became permanent.)

• The medical literature contains reports of patients exhibiting symptoms of multiple sclerosis due to a deficiency of R binder, a protein that plays an essential role in B$_{12}$ metabolism.

All of these facts hint that MS and B$_{12}$ deficiency may somehow be intertwined. Unfortunately, only a minority of patients with true MS improve appreciably when they receive injections of vitamin B$_{12}$—although this disappointing result could possibly be influenced by the form of B$_{12}$ they are given (see Chapter 11).

To clarify the possible B$_{12}$–MS link, scientists are now focusing on the following two questions:

1. *Does B$_{12}$ deficiency contribute to the development of MS?* Research shows that people who develop multiple sclerosis before the age of eighteen have lower B$_{12}$ levels than those who develop MS in adulthood. Because B$_{12}$ levels are unrelated to the length of the illness, researchers say, "these findings suggest a specific association between the timing of onset of the first neurological symptoms of MS and vitamin B$_{12}$ metabolism."[15] They speculate that B$_{12}$ deficiency—which suppresses the immune system's ability to fight off viruses and bacteria—could leave some people more vulnerable to MS by impairing their defenses against the infections that are widely suspected of playing a role in the genesis of MS.

2. *Does B$_{12}$ deficiency make it harder for the body to repair the myelin damage that occurs in MS?* Vitamin B$_{12}$ plays a crucial role in

myelin formation, and research suggests that the body may require normal or even higher-than-normal levels of B$_{12}$ in order to reverse the myelin damage caused by MS.[16] If so, MS patients with low levels of B$_{12}$ may be less likely to go into remission.

All of these findings are very preliminary, and we don't yet know if B$_{12}$ deficiency puts people at increased risk for MS, or whether it inhibits their ability to go into remission once they have the disease. However, researchers should focus on finding answers to these questions. Few diseases strike the young and healthy with as much cruelty as MS, and if it turns out that B$_{12}$ can play some role in protecting against the disease, or in improving its course when it occurs, this knowledge could be invaluable to thousands of MS patients.

In the meantime, we urge that any MS patient, *with or without signs of B$_{12}$ deficiency*, should first be tested and then start a long-term trial of injectable B$_{12}$. We recommend a B$_{12}$ trial even if the tests are negative for a deficiency, because we don't yet fully understand the connection between MS and B$_{12}$ metabolism.

We are aware that this is not standard practice for most physicians who treat MS. However, vitamin B$_{12}$ is nontoxic, even in high doses, so it's risk-free except for patients with a very rare condition called Leber's disease (see Chapter 11), and a small, but significant, percentage of MS patients report that treatment makes them significantly better. In some cases, the improvement is dramatic, and occasionally it occurs even after years of disability. Thus, to our way of thinking, it makes sense—given the lack of a "down side"—for every MS patient to give B$_{12}$ a chance.

Is It Multiple Sclerosis or B_{12} Deficiency—or Both?

If you're experiencing symptoms that resemble multiple sclerosis, or if you have already been diagnosed with MS, your doctor needs to order the following tests in order to rule out B_{12} deficiency. Defects in B_{12} utilization stemming from inborn errors of B_{12} metabolism or transport are difficult to detect without tests more sensitive than a serum B_{12} test. If your doctor questions the need for any of these tests, refer him or her to Chapter 11:

1. Urine or serum methylmalonic acid (MMA)
   a. Lab must use gas chromatography/mass spectrometry (GC/MS) technique
   b. Urine must be used if patient has renal insufficiency/dehydration/recent history of antibiotic use
2. Serum B_{12}
3. Plasma homocysteine (Hcy)

If any of the above tests come back borderline or positive, your doctor needs to order the following additional blood tests, and he or she should start you on hydroxocobalamin or methylcobalamin injections (see Chapter 11):

1. Parietal cell antibody
2. Intrinsic factor antibody
3. Gastrin (twelve-hour fast required)
4. Unsaturated B_{12}-binding capacity (serum)

Note: If possible, your doctor should order these tests before beginning any treatment with steroids, Copaxone, Betaseron, or Avonex (Rebif). It is unknown if treatment with these drugs can alter the results of MMA and/or homocysteine tests. Also, testing should be done before you try any nutritional or homeopathic interventions, which may skew the test results.

Notes

1. Roach, E. Steve, and McLean, William T. Neurologic disorders of B12 deficiency. *American Family Physician*, 1982, 25:111–115.
2. Heath, Thomas. Pernicious anemia: One man's journey through the baffling world of medical diagnosis. *Washington Post*, February 22, 2000, p. Z–12.
3. Schilling, R. F., and Williams, W. J. Vitamin B12 deficiency: Underdiagnosed, overtreated? *Hospital Practice*, July 15, 1995, 47–54.
4. Wilhelm, H., Grodd, W., Schiefer, U., and Zrenner, E. Uncommon chiasmal lesions: demyelinating disease, vasculitis, and cobalamin deficiency. *German Journal of Ophthalmology* 1993, 2:234–40.
5. Hotchkiss, J. Vitamin B$_{12}$—A Controversial Vitamin (conference presentation). June 2001, Society for Orthomolecular Medicine, San Francisco.
6. Carmel, R., Watkins, D., Goodman, S. I., and Rosenblatt, D. S. Hereditary defect of cobalamin metabolism (cblG mutation) presenting as a neurologic disorder in adulthood. *New England Journal of Medicine* 1988, 318(26):1738–41.
7. Trojano, M., and Paolicelli, D. The differential diagnosis of multiple sclerosis: Classification and clinical features of relapsing and progressive neurological syndromes. *Neurological Sciences* 2001 Suppl 2:S98–102.
8. Schilling, R. F., and Williams, W. J. Vitamin B$_{12}$ deficiency: Underdiagnosed, overtreated? *Hospital Practice*, July 15, 1995, 47–54.
9. Ibid.
10. Norman, E. J. Cobalamin (vitamin B$_{12}$) deficiency identified in young, Caucasian women. *Blood*, 2000, 96(11):8b.
11. Payinda, G., and Hansen, T. Vitamin B(12) deficiency manifested as psychosis without anemia. *American Journal of Psychiatry* 2000, 157:660–61.
12. Physician information posted on the Neurology and Neurosurgery Forum, in answer to a question. Questions on the forum are answered by physicians from the Cleveland Clinic, a major U.S. hospital.
13. Goodkin, D. E., et al. Serum cobalamin deficiency is uncommon in multiple sclerosis. *Archives of Neurology* 1994, 51:1110–14.
14. Kira, Jun-ichi, Tobimatsu, Shozo, and Goto, Ikuo. Vitamin B$_{12}$ metabolism and massive-dose methyl vitamin B$_{12}$ therapy in Japanese patients with multiple sclerosis. *Internal Medicine* 1994, 33:82–86.
15. Sandyk, R., and Awerbuch, G. I. Vitamin B$_{12}$ and its relationship to age of onset of multiple sclerosis. *International Journal of Neuroscience* (England) Jul–Aug 1993, 71: p93–9.
16. Kira, J., Tobimatsu, S., and Goto, I. Vitamin B$_{12}$ metabolism and massive-dose methyl vitamin B$_{12}$ therapy in Japanese patients with multiple sclerosis. *Internal Medicine* 1994, 33:82–86.

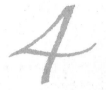

Am I Losing My Mind? When B_{12} Deficiency Causes Mental Illness

"Deficiency of essential nutrients like folic acid and vitamin B_{12} is an obvious risk factor for both disorders with cognitive impairment and depression." —C. G. Gottfries, M.D.[1]

"Current research suggests that low levels of vitamin B_{12} are associated with dementia and depression.... Vitamin B_{12} deficiency has also been associated with psychosis, bipolar disorder, and catatonia."
—Psychiatrist Glenn Catalano, M.D., and colleagues[2]

"I have gained a distinct sense that we physicians, neurologists, and psychiatrists have been miserly with our B_{12} diagnoses and treatments." —John Dommisse, M.D.[3]

In the last chapter, we explained how B_{12} deficiency attacks the nerves, stripping them of their protective myelin coating and disrupting the communication between cells in the brain and other parts of the nervous system. This damage, as we noted, can make you lose your balance, develop multiple sclerosis-like symptoms, or suffer shooting pains or numbness in your feet, hands, arms, or legs. It can also make your memory fuzzy, and even mimic Alzheimer's disease.

But the damage that B_{12} depletion causes can affect your nervous system in other ways as well. Because the nerve cells in your brain control how you feel, think, and behave, B_{12} deficiency can cause severe mental illness, including depression, paranoia, and even symptoms resembling schizophrenia. A deficiency of B$_{12}$ is not the cause of *most* cases of mental illness, but it clearly plays a powerful role in a number of cases—and particularly in cases involving depression or bipolar disorder (manic depression).

The middle-aged man had been happy and healthy most of his life, but some time after his fiftieth birthday his behavior changed radically. He became hyperactive, and he no longer slept more than a few hours each night. Worse, he developed the strange flights of thought and grandiose ideas typical of people in the manic phase of bipolar disorder.

After four years, however, the man began suffering very different symptoms: He became anxious and sad, stopped eating, and was tired all the time. Eventually, he began having paranoid thoughts about his wife.

Finally, the man encountered a new physician who checked his B$_{12}$ levels—which were so low that his plasma B$_{12}$ was "undetectable." Further tests revealed that he had pernicious anemia [autoimmune disease], and the new doctor started him on regular B$_{12}$ shots.

"His mental state improved dramatically within a few days," physicians P. M. Verbanck and O. LeBon report in the Journal of Clinical Psychiatry. *"By the end of the first week of treatment, the only remaining symptom was the paranoid delusions." These slowly subsided, disappearing completely after six months of treatment.*[4]

The patient described above had bipolar disorder because his B$_{12}$ levels were so low that his brain couldn't function correctly. In his case, the problem stemmed from pernicious anemia, but people with dangerously low B$_{12}$ due to other causes are equally at risk of developing severe depression or bipolar disorder.

How dramatically can B$_{12}$ deficiency increase your risk of developing severe, life-threatening depression? Researchers at the National Institute on Aging, evaluating a group of disabled women over the age of sixty-five, found that B$_{12}$ deficiency *doubled* the risk of severe depression in this group. The researchers, noting that these were independent women living in the community, report, "It should be an alarming sign that we found [a significant rate of B$_{12}$-deficiency-caused depression] in this population."[5]

In a related study, Dutch researchers screened nearly four thousand older individuals for depression, and then compared the laboratory tests results of those with depressive symptoms to non-depressed control group members. The researchers report that high homocysteine levels, vitamin B$_{12}$ deficiency, and to a lesser extent, folate deficiency were all related to depressive disorders. When they controlled for other factors, the effects of homocysteine and folic acid levels were less prominent, but low B$_{12}$ levels were still strongly associated with depression.[6]

People over sixty are at the highest risk for depression due to B$_{12}$ deficiency, but anyone, at any age, can be a victim. Moreover, B$_{12}$ deficiency appears to put individuals at especially high risk for psychotic depression, which involves terrifying symptoms, such as hallucinations and paranoia. Researchers evaluating fifty-three patients suffering from major depression found that the average B$_{12}$ concentration of those with psychotic depression was very low (below 182 pg/ml, indicating deficiency), while those with non-psychotic depression had more normal results.[7]

Because psychotic depression so often drives its victims to commit murder or suicide, it's particularly critical that doctors check any depressed patients with symptoms of psychosis for low B$_{12}$. Prompt treatment of psychotic depression stemming from B$_{12}$ deficiency can lead to almost immediate recovery, even in the most severe cases.

Two young Bedouin women, brought to an Israeli hospital at different times, were experiencing terrible hallucinations. One, an eighteen-year-old, believed that a giant, hideous monster was trying to strangle her. The other, a twenty-three-year-old, heard threatening voices and suffered both daytime and nighttime hallucinations involving human figures trying to hurt her. Both women were depressed, anxious, and suffering from a severe lack of sleep. They'd been treated with antipsychotic drugs, but the medications didn't work.

Doctors at Ben-Gurion University measured the women's B$_{12}$ levels and found that both were profoundly deficient. Interestingly, neither showed the blood abnormalities typical of B$_{12}$ deficiency, apparently because both ate diets rich in folic acid (which, as we've explained, can mask the blood signs of low B$_{12}$).

The doctors started both women on injected B$_{12}$. One recovered completely within six weeks, and the other within eight weeks. Both are now taking daily high-dose oral supplements of B$_{12}$ and have no symptoms one year later.

The doctors report, "Although these women were not vegetarians, dietary analysis showed that their daily diet was based predominantly on bread, vegetables, and canned food, with a minimal intake of meat or dairy products."[8] *This diet is very similar in B$_{12}$ content to that consumed by many American vegetarians and vegans who forgo meat and dairy products and to that of many dieters who follow diets that limit meat, milk, and cheese.*

Depression, however, isn't the only mental illness that B$_{12}$ deficiency can cause. As we noted in Chapter 2, it can cause dementia as well, and research and case studies reported in the literature show that B$_{12}$ deficiency can also lead to delusions, hallucinations and other schizophrenia-like symptoms, obsessive-compulsive symptoms, and a wide range of other psychiatric problems. The following is a sampling of cases taken from medical journals:

- Physician G. Daynes reported, many years ago, that in his own practice as medical director of a hospital in South Africa, he successfully treated eight women whose postpartum psychosis stemmed from B$_{12}$ deficiency. (Postpartum psychosis is the disorder involved in the well-publicized case of Andrea Yates, who murdered her five children, and it is linked to many other suicides and murders.) His patients' recoveries led him to recommend that all women with postpartum psychosis receive large doses of B$_{12}$. "Where the postpartum psychosis is not primarily caused by lack of vitamin B$_{12}$, the giving of the preparation will do no harm," he noted, "so it seems to me that in all such cases it should be given as soon as possible."[9]
- Doctors in Australia, evaluating a patient diagnosed with anxiety disorder and conversion disorder—a psychiatric diagnosis applied when doctors believe that a patient is converting emotional distress into physical symptoms, such as paralysis or blindness—discovered that she didn't have a psychiatric illness at all. She had a physical illness, B$_{12}$ deficiency, caused by her illegal use of "whipped cream bulbs," containing nitrous oxide (a popular recreational drug—see Chapter 8). When the doctors gave her three injections of B$_{12}$, her

mental and physical symptoms disappeared almost completely.[10] This case illustrates the need for doctors to screen all young people with psychiatric symptoms or suspected histories of drug abuse for B$_{12}$ deficiency.

• Doctors in Massachusetts, treating a twenty-year-old woman who'd attempted suicide three months earlier, discovered the reason for the woman's urges to kill herself: She had autoimmune pernicious anemia. She now receives regular injections of B$_{12}$, which have eliminated her depression and suicidal thoughts.[11]

• Dr. Frederick Goggans and colleagues reported the case of an elderly man who suddenly developed severe mania, believing that his hometown was planning a large celebration in his honor, including appearances by Hollywood celebrities. "He became so physically energized," the doctors noted, "that six younger men were required to restrain him at the time of admission to the hospital." Lab tests showed a drastically low B$_{12}$ level, and his doctors eventually diagnosed pernicious anemia and treated him with B$_{12}$ injections. He recovered quickly, and at his six-month checkup he was doing fine.[12]

Routine B$_{12}$ screening of psychiatric patients could help to identify people like these, well before their declining B$_{12}$ levels lead to mental illness—and there are far more such people than doctors realize. In one recent study, researchers measured the serum B$_{12}$ levels of patients admitted to a general hospital and exhibiting psychiatric symptoms. (It should be noted that the researchers *excluded* all patients already diagnosed with B$_{12}$ deficiency.) They divided the patients into three categories—those with normal/high B$_{12}$, those with levels below 400 pg/mL (a level many researchers suggest should be the minimum), and those with levels lower than 200 pg/mL (the level the United States considers the acceptable threshold for serum B$_{12}$, although this number almost undoubtedly is far too low).

Of the 115 patients with depression or other mood disorders, the researchers reported, nearly a third had B$_{12}$ levels below the first cutoff point of 400 pg/mL, and seven had levels below 200, indicating overt

Tests that Could Save a Mother's Sanity —and a Child's Life

More research is needed to determine the incidence of B$_{12}$ deficiency in women with postpartum depression or postpartum psychosis. In the meantime, we believe that all women diagnosed with postpartum mental illness should undergo screening, including serum B$_{12}$, urinary MMA, and Hcy tests. Pregnancy can dramatically worsen a pre-existing B$_{12}$ deficiency, because B$_{12}$ is transferred to the growing fetus throughout pregnancy, and prenatal vitamins contain only six micrograms of this nutrient (compared to the 1,000 micrograms needed to treat a deficiency). Pregnant women at greatest risk for deficiency include vegans and vegetarians, those with autoimmune pernicious anemia or malabsorption syndromes such as Crohn's disease (an inflammatory intestinal disease) or celiac disease, and those with a history of strict dieting, anorexia, or bulimia. However, any woman who develops symptoms of mental illness following pregnancy needs B$_{12}$ screening. It is crucial for doctors to identify the root causes of postpartum depression or psychosis—causes that appear to include B$_{12}$ deficiency in some cases—because, as the tragic case of Andrea Yates shows, more than one life may be at stake.

deficiency. Of the thirty-four patients with cognitive spectrum disorders, one-fifth had levels below 400 pg/mL, and two had levels below 200.

The researchers note that "the societal costs of mood disorders and cognitive disorders are staggering," with depression treatment alone costing nearly 44 billion dollars annually in the United States, and they say that given the inexpensiveness of testing patients for B$_{12}$ or folate deficiency, "Our findings do support the need for early identification of vitamin B$_{12}$ and folate deficiencies before clinically significant physical and mental symptoms appear."[13]

In another recent study, researchers reviewed laboratory data from psychiatric patients, and they also measured B$_{12}$ levels in a random sampling of patients whose dietary habits were documented. They report that 20 percent of the patients had serum vitamin B$_{12}$ levels below 200 pg/

mL, and 10 percent had levels below 160 pg/mL, indicating severe deficiency. "Our findings confirm that vitamin B$_{12}$ deficiency is not uncommon in psychiatric patients, even when exposed to adequate nutrition," they conclude, adding, "The true prevalence may be even greater since low serum levels may underestimate the actual extent of vitamin B$_{12}$ deficiency."[14] Similarly, when Dr. H. Hermesh and colleagues studied thirty patients with obsessive-compulsive disorder, they found that 20 percent of them had abnormally low levels of B$_{12}$.[15]

When did doctors discover the link between B$_{12}$ and mental illness?

The answer is, over a century ago—which makes it all the more surprising that most doctors fail to routinely consider B$_{12}$ deficiency as a cause of psychiatric patients' symptoms.

Physicians Melvin Hector and John Burton note in a journal article[16] that in the early 1900s, doctors discovered that pernicious anemia (one form of B$_{12}$ deficiency) caused symptoms including apathy, decreased ability to do mental work, loss of memory, restlessness, irritability, indifference, emotional instability, disorientation and confusion, loss of inhibition, dementia, delirium, depression, delusions and hallucinations, confabulation, hysteria, neurasthenia, paranoia, and mania. These psychiatric manifestations were termed "megaloblastic madness," because people who had enlarged red blood cells (macrocytosis) caused by B$_{12}$ deficiency often appeared to have gone "mad."

In the late 1920s, when doctors first learned to treat pernicious anemia by giving patients large amounts of raw liver, multiple case reports showed that these very same psychiatric symptoms abated in treated patients. Similar reports of psychiatric symptoms caused by deficient B$_{12}$, and successfully treated by administering the vitamin, appeared on a regular basis over the remainder of the 1900s. Yet at the turn of a new century, when we have the benefit of nearly a hundred years of research showing a connection between B$_{12}$ deficiency and psychiatric illness, not all mentally ill patients are being evaluated for underlying B$_{12}$ deficiency—and only a small percentage receive the adjunctive urinary MMA test that will reveal deficiency, even when serum B$_{12}$ and complete blood count tests are normal.

As a nursing school project, one of us (Sally) once analyzed psychiatrists' patterns of testing for B$_{12}$ deficiency in a psychiatric facility.

Of thirty-one inpatients seen during this study, only seven received se-rum B12 tests, and *no* patients under the age of sixty were tested. Eight of the patients exhibited blood smear evidence of B$_{12}$ deficiency, but none of these patients' doctors ordered serum B$_{12}$ tests. One paranoid and demented patient who finally received testing, and proved to be dras-tically deficient in B$_{12}$, had been admitted to the same facility the previ-ous year for the same symptoms, but had been discharged without doc-tors ever suspecting the cause of his problems. By the time he received a diagnosis during his second visit, it was too late to help him. He'd lived for a year in a nursing home after his first visit, when doctors described him as having "paranoid psychosis with dementia and multi-infarct de-mentia"—an accurate label, but one that did nothing to explain why he suffered from psychosis and dementia, or to correct the problem before it became irreversible.

The cost of such oversights, in terms of human suffering, is inesti-mable. The cost in health-care dollars is significant as well. Compare, for instance, the cost of B$_{12}$ treatment (which, as we've noted, averages about fifteen dollars per year) to the cost of the commonly prescribed psychiatric drugs Ativan ($677 per year), Paxil ($1,220 per year), Prozac ($2,243 per year), or Risperdal ($3,525 per year)—not to mention the cost of psychiatric admissions or repeated emergency room visits.

The woman who came to our emergency department complaining of abdominal bloating and spine pain had a reputation with her doctors. Some thought she was crazy. Others labeled her as a drug-seeker, faking mental and physical illnesses in order to get prescriptions for drugs.

Her medical record, however, told a far different story. She'd under-gone bypass surgery for weight-loss fifteen years earlier, impairing her body's ability to obtain B$_{12}$. Her medical records contained four years worth of lab tests, showing enlarged blood cells, a classic sign of B$_{12}$ deficiency. She'd been through numerous surgeries, many of them no doubt involving nitrous oxide, which can destroy B$_{12}$ stores (see Chapter 8). She had a history of hypothyroidism, often found in association with au-toimmune pernicious anemia. Her neurological and psychiatric symp-toms—poor balance, spinal pain, gait abnormalities, anxiety—are text-book symptoms of a deficiency of B$_{12}$.

This sad and frightened woman had seen thirteen doctors, and not one identified her real problem. Some merely placed her on multivitamin *and folic acid supplements, assuming that her enlarged blood cells stemmed from folic acid deficiency due to a poor diet or alcoholism. Others dismissed her problems as "all in her head." And, all left her in agonizing pain, both mental and physical, and forced her to continue her search for a drug or doctor capable of saving her from her misery. Our emergency department staff finally did save her, by testing her B$_{12}$ level. It was 146 pg/ml, a level low enough to explain all of the symptoms that had ruined her life for more than a decade.*

In addition to causing mental illness in people with no history of psychiatric disease, B$_{12}$ deficiency can cause a dramatic worsening of symptoms in people already diagnosed with mental disorders. Often, doctors dismiss these worsening symptoms as "just another phase" of the existing condition, or they treat them with ever-heavier doses of psychiatric drugs that do nothing at all to treat depleted B$_{12}$ levels.

If you've been diagnosed with any mental disorder, or your symptoms suddenly become much worse or return after a period of remission, it's important to rule out B$_{12}$ deficiency as a cause—*even if your doctors say that B$_{12}$ has nothing to do with your preexisting illness.* As psychiatrist Sydney Walker once noted, "Having one illness doesn't protect you from having another." In fact, mental disorders can make you more vulnerable to B$_{12}$ deficiency, because they increase the odds that you're eating poorly, or taking drugs that can compromise your B$_{12}$ metabolism.

If your new symptoms do stem from a B$_{12}$ problem, treating these symptoms with psychiatric drugs will simply allow the damage to your brain and nervous system to continue, with possibly fatal consequences. Correcting this deficiency, conversely, can often result in prompt and dramatic improvement.

Some psychiatric patients are lucky to have doctors who look for root causes when new symptoms arise. One was a middle-aged man who'd suffered a head injury decades earlier, resulting in behavior changes that his doctors successfully controlled with medication.

One day, the man suddenly became lethargic and began slurring his speech. By the time his caregivers brought him to the emergency department, he was in a stupor, exhibiting depression and oddly slowed movements, a mask-like flat expression, and abnormally slow speech.

Diagnosing him as catatonic, his doctors could have assumed that *his problems stemmed from his earlier head injury and simply added more drugs to his treatment plan—or admitted him to a psychiatric hospital, where he might have languished for the rest of his life. Instead, they ran tests, discovered that he was severely B$_{12}$ deficient, and they treated him with B$_{12}$ injections.*

After two weeks in the hospital, they reported, the man "was speaking spontaneously in sentences, had a wide emotional range, and was interacting with the other patients.... He was able to ambulate on his own, with improved balance and coordination.... There were no psychotic or depressive symptoms seen."[17]

In a similar case reported by different doctors, a schizophrenic man who'd been in remission for four years began displaying psychotic symptoms after a bout of pneumonia. His doctors could have said, "It's just a relapse." Instead, they tested his B$_{12}$ levels, which proved to be low. Within five days of B$_{12}$ therapy, the man's symptoms disappeared and he could once again lead a normal life.[18]

Taking the lead in getting tested

The medical profession underestimates the role of B$_{12}$ deficiency in mental illness, rarely suspecting this disorder in patients with depression, anxiety, bipolar disorder, or other psychiatric problems. So, if you suffer from psychiatric symptoms, or you're caring for a spouse, child, or other loved one with a mental illness, it's up to you to insist on thorough B$_{12}$ testing.

If your psychiatrist is reluctant to test you or your loved one, it may be necessary to consult other doctors, including your family physician or other specialists, in order to find one who is willing to order the tests. (Conversely, we sometimes find that psychiatrists are more willing than other doctors to order B$_{12}$ testing. For instance, the fifty-one-year-old woman we discussed in the previous chapter—who was diagnosed with multiple sclerosis, and eventually developed severe mental illness and tried to throw herself out of a moving car—received her diagnosis from a psychiatrist, after her other specialists missed the call.) When you do find a doctor who agrees to evaluate you or a loved one for B$_{12}$ deficiency, make sure the tests include a serum B$_{12}$ level, a urinary MMA, and a plasma homocysteine (see chapters 10 and 11). Do *not* assume that a doctor will order these tests, because they are not part of most standard psychiatric evaluations.

Be assertive in insisting on these tests, and be sure that you get treatment—lifelong treatment, when necessary—if a deficiency is detected. We see far too many patients who've suffered unnecessarily for months or years, when a few tests and a shot of B$_{12}$ every month could have cured their psychiatric symptoms completely. With your own sanity, or the well-being of a loved one at stake, why take a chance?

Psychiatric Symptoms that Can Be Associated with B$_{12}$ Deficiency

Note: A number of these symptoms overlap with dementia, which we discuss in Chapter 2.

Among the most common psychiatric symptoms seen in people with B$_{12}$ deficiency are the following:

- confusion/disorientation
- memory loss
- depression
- mania
- paranoia
- irritability
- apathy
- personality changes
- inappropriate sexual behavior
- delusions
- hallucinations
- violent/aggressive behavior
- schizophrenic symptoms
- sleep disturbances
- changes in taste, smell, vision, and sensory/ motor function that can be mistaken for psychiatric problems

Notes

1. Gottfries, C. G. Late life depression. *European Archives of Psychiatry and Clinical Neuroscience* 2001, 251(Suppl 2):57–61.
2. Catalano, G., Catalano, M. C., O'Dell, K. J., Humphrey, D. A., and Fritz, E. B. The utility of laboratory screening in medically ill patients with psychiatric symptoms. *Annals of Clinical Psychiatry* 2001, 13(3):135–140.
3. Dommisse, J. Letter re "Case report: The psychiatric manifestation of B$_{12}$ deficiency." *Primary Psychiatry* 1996, 3(1):50–5. Cited at www.johndommissemd.com.
4. Verbanck, P., and LeBon, O. Changing psychiatric symptoms in a patient with vitamin B$_{12}$ deficiency. *Journal of Clinical Psychiatry* 1991, 52(4):182–3.
5. Penninx, B. W., et al. Vitamin B$_{12}$ deficiency and depression in physically disabled older women: Epidemiologic evidence from the Women's Health and Aging Study. *American Journal of Psychiatry* 2000 May;157(5):715–21.
6. Tiemeier, H., van Tuijl, H. R., Hofman, A., Meijer, J., Kiliaan, A. J., and Breteler, M. M. Vitamin B$_{12}$, folate, and homocysteine in depression: The Rotterdam Study. *American Journal of Psychiatry* 2002, 159(12):2099–101.
7. Levitt, A., and Joffe, R. Vitamin B$_{12}$ in psychotic depression. *British Journal of Psychiatry* 1988, 153:266–7.
8. Masalha, R., Chudakov, B., Muhamad, M., Rudoy, I., Volkov, I., and Wirguin, I. Cobalamin-responsive psychosis as the sole manifestation of vitamin B$_{12}$ deficiency. *Israeli Medical Association Journal* 2001, 3:701–3.
9. Daynes, G. Cyanocobalamin in postpartum psychosis. *South African Medical Journal* 1975, 49(34):1373.
10. Brett, A. Myeloneuropathy from whipped cream bulbs presenting as conversion disorder. *Australia and New Zealand Journal of Psychiatry* 1997, 31(1):131–2.
11. Middleman, A. B., and Melchiono, M. W. A routine CBC leads to a non-routine diagnosis. *Adolescent Medicine* 1996, 7(3):423–6.
12. Goggans, F. C. A case of mania secondary to vitamin B$_{12}$ deficiency. *American Journal of Psychiatry* 1984, 141(2):300–1.
13. Catalano, G., Catalano, M. C., O'Dell, K. J., Humphrey, D. A., and Fritz, E. B. The utility of laboratory screening in medically ill patients with psychiatric symptoms. *Annals of Clinical Psychiatry* 2001, 13(3):135–140.
14. Silver, H. Vitamin B$_{12}$ levels are low in hospitalized psychiatric patients. *Israeli Journal of Psychiatry and Related Sciences* 2000, 37(1):41–5.
15. Hermesh, H., Weizman, A., Shahar, A., and Munitz, H. Vitamin B$_{12}$ and folic acid serum levels in obsessive compulsive disorder. *Acta Psychiatrica Scandinavia* 1988, 78(1):8–10.
16. Hector, M., and Burton, J. What are the psychiatric manifestations of

vitamin B$_{12}$ deficiency? *Journal of the American Geriatric Society* 1988, 36:1105-12.

17. Catalano, G., Catalano, M. C., Roenberg, E. I., Embi, P. J., and Embi, C. S. Catatonia: Another neuropsychiatric presentation of vitamin B$_{12}$ deficiency? *Psychosomatics* 1998, 39(5):456.

18. Buchman, N., Mendelsson, E., Lerner, V., and Kotler, M. Delirium associated with vitamin B$_{12}$ deficiency after pneumonia. *Clinical Neuropharmacology* 1999, 22(6):356–8.

5

Stroke, Heart Disease, and Other Vascular Problems: The B_{12}-Homocysteine Connection

"High homocysteine can increase the risk of heart attack as much as high cholesterol." —Abbott Laboratories[1]

Scientists investigating the causes of cardiovascular disease are zeroing in on one culprit in particular—a risk identified more than thirty years ago, but ignored by doctors until recently. It's homocysteine, an amino acid that can wreak havoc on your cardiovascular system. High homocysteine levels put you at risk for coronary artery disease, heart attacks, strokes, deep vein thromboses (blood clots), and other deadly vascular problems. In fact, homocysteine has been dubbed "the cholesterol of the next century."[2]

What does this have to do with vitamin B_{12}? A great deal, because B_{12} allows another nutrient, folic acid, to convert homocysteine into a nontoxic amino acid. When your B_{12} levels drop to unhealthy levels, this process breaks down, and your homocysteine levels rise sharply—along with your risk of heart attack or stroke.

What is homocysteine and why is it so bad for you?

The story of homocysteine begins with the food you eat. That food contains twenty amino acids, one of which is methionine.

Your body breaks down methionine into smaller particles, one of which is a molecule called SAMe. SAMe, in turn, breaks down into smaller substances, one of which is homocysteine. When everything's working right, this homocysteine quickly gets recycled back into methionine with the help of vitamin B_{12} and folic acid, following two pathways (see below). Any excess homocysteine winds up in your liver, which breaks it down with the help of vitamins B_{12}, B_6, and folic acid. But if you're deficient in any one of these vitamins, this normal cycle is disrupted and homocysteine accumulates in your blood, with no place to go.

That's dangerous, because homocysteine, while it's a "good guy" when it's rapidly transformed into beneficial substances, is a "bad guy" when left on its own. Excess homocysteine causes your blood vessels to lose their elasticity, making it harder for them to dilate, and damaging their inner lining. That damage, in turn, allows cholesterol, collagen, and

Homocysteine Recycling Pathways

The following are the two pathways that continuously recycle homocysteine (Hcy) back into methionine:

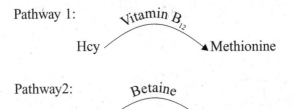

Pathway 1:

Vitamin B_{12}

Hcy → Methionine

Pathway2:

Betaine

Hcy → Methionine

When B_{12} deficiency is present, Hcy will rise and methionine will decrease.

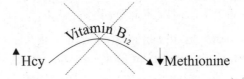

Vitamin B_{12}

↑Hcy → ↓Methionine

The recycling of homocysteine is important for the building of thousands of compounds and proteins that are necessary for healthy cells, tissues, and organs. Homocysteine is also detoxified and made harmless through a process called transsulfuration, which requires B_6, magnesium, and SAMe.

calcium to attach to the inner walls of your blood vessels, where they can form sticky deposits called atherosclerotic plaques. These plaques narrow your arteries, and drastically increase your risk of suffering deadly disorders, such as coronary artery disease, heart attacks, strokes, "mini strokes" (transient ischemic attacks, or TIAs), blood clots, carotid and renal artery stenosis (narrowing), or aneurysms (ballooning of damaged blood vessels). In addition, elevated homocysteine levels alter your biochemistry in ways that appear to promote abnormal blood clotting.[3]

Homocysteine is also an "oxidant" that decreases the production of nitric oxide*—a substance crucial to healthy blood vessel function. Decreased nitric oxide, in turn, is strongly linked to both atherosclerosis and high blood pressure.

Initially, researchers wondered if high homocysteine, rather than causing cardiovascular disease, simply occurred as a side effect. Studies show, however, that elevated homocysteine *precedes* the onset of disease.[4] This strongly indicates that homocysteine, rather than just being a marker for cardiovascular disease, actively contributes to the disease process.

Five to 10 percent of the population, and as many as 30 to 40 percent of senior citizens, have elevated homocysteine levels.[5] The older you are, the more likely you are to have high homocysteine. Men tend to have higher levels than women, smokers often have higher levels than nonsmokers, and genes play a major role in influencing your homocysteine level. Certain medications, too, can affect homocysteine status, as can impaired kidney function. But in people without kidney problems, the primary cause of the problem, no matter what other factors are involved, is a low level of folate and/or vitamin B$_{12}$, or, to a lesser degree, a low level of vitamin B$_6$.

Why folate can't do the job by itself

Increasing numbers of doctors are aware of the dangers of high homocysteine, and of the benefits of folic acid therapy. Unfortunately, few of these doctors fully understand the critical role that vitamin B$_{12}$ plays in detoxifying homocysteine. This is a serious oversight, because people with high homocysteine levels often respond fully *only* when they're given large amounts of B$_{12}$ as well. The reason: People who are deficient in B$_{12}$

---

*Nitric oxide, by the way, should not be confused with the anesthetic agent nitrous oxide. The two names sound alike, but there is no relationship.

can't assimilate folic acid properly, and as a result, much of the folic acid is trapped in an inaccessible form. Thus, testing for B_{12} deficiency (and treatment if needed) must always be part of a homocysteine-lowering program.

Yet, many cardiologists prescribe only folic acid to patients with high homocysteine levels, and many others merely augment this folic acid regimen with a multivitamin containing small amounts of B_{12}. This is often ineffective, because a few micrograms of B_{12} won't correct a significant deficiency. If you have high homocysteine levels, your doctor needs to determine if a vitamin B_{12} deficiency exists, by testing both your serum B_{12} level and your urinary MMA (see Chapter 10). Proper treatment of high homocysteine may include high doses of both folic acid and vitamin B_{12}, and if you have a B_{12} deficiency due to a malabsorption or autoimmune problem, your treatment may need to include B_{12} injections instead of oral therapy.

A powerful connection

How strong is the link between high homocysteine and cardiovascular disease? Israeli researchers recently decided to find out, by comparing the homocysteine levels of people whose fathers had suffered heart attacks to the levels of people whose fathers had no such history. In addition, the researchers compared homocysteine levels of people in Jerusalem, where the rate of heart attacks is high, with the levels of people in the United States, where the heart attack rate is lower.

The researchers found that male children of heart attack victims had significantly higher homocysteine levels than control group members. When they charted the homocysteine levels of all of the study subjects, they found that people in the top 20 percent were far more likely than other subjects to be in the "parental heart attack" group.

In addition, men in Jerusalem had much higher homocysteine levels than the U.S. men—a logical explanation for their higher heart attack rate. The researchers add that the difference in homocysteine levels between men in the two countries "was largely attributable to *lower plasma vitamin B_{12} levels* [emphasis added] in the Israeli population."[6]

In a different study, conducted as part of the prestigious large-scale Physicians' Health Study, researchers compared doctors who'd suffered heart attacks during a five-year period to those with healthy hearts. The researchers analyzed homocysteine levels using plasma samples the doctors donated at the beginning of the study.

After controlling for age and smoking habits, the researchers reported, "Moderately high levels of plasma homocysteine are associated with subsequent risk of myocardial infarction [heart attack] independent of other coronary risk factors." Men in the top 5 percent of homocysteine level were more than three times as likely as other subjects to suffer heart attacks. The researchers concluded, "Because high levels can often be easily treated with vitamin supplements, homocysteine may be an independent, modifiable risk factor."[7]

Even more dramatic findings appeared in the *New England Journal of Medicine* a few years ago. Norwegian researchers followed 587 patients with existing coronary artery disease. Within about five years of undergoing treatment, 11 percent of the patients had died. "We found a strong, graded relation between plasma homocysteine levels and overall mortality," the researchers reported, with around 4 percent of patients in the low-homocysteine group dying as compared to nearly one quarter of those in the high-homocysteine group. The strong correlation remained even after the researchers controlled for other risk factors.

"Our results," the researchers said, "should serve as an additional strong incentive to the initiation of intervention trials with homocysteine-lowering therapy."[8] So should similar results from a recent study of more than 400 patients who'd suffered heart attacks or unstable angina. In this study, the long-term death rate from cardiac disease was more than twice as high for patients in the upper two quintiles of homocysteine level as it was for other patients.[9]

Still more evidence comes from a recent "meta-analysis"—a study that pools data from multiple studies in order to increase statistical power. Physician David Wald and colleagues evaluated seventy-two genetic studies analyzing the effects of a common gene variant that raises homocysteine levels, as well as twenty prospective studies analyzing the association between serum homocysteine levels and disease risk. "The genetic studies and the prospective studies do not share the same potential sources of error, but both yield similarly highly significant results—strong evidence that the association between homocysteine and cardiovascular disease is causal," the researchers concluded.[10]

Even in young people, research shows high homocysteine is a threat. A recent large-scale study found that elevated homocysteine nearly doubles the risk of stroke in women between the ages of fifteen and forty-four. Said the researchers, "The magnitude of the increase in stroke risk was similar to that of smoking a pack of cigarettes per day."[11]

Dozens of additional studies corroborate these findings, implicating high homocysteine as one of the most powerful cardiovascular risk factors ever identified. Luckily, it's a problem that is easy to treat—and the treatment begins by lowering homocysteine levels almost immediately. One recent study, lasting only eight weeks, tested the effects of folic acid alone, B_{12} alone, and folic acid plus B_{12} in lowering the homocysteine levels of patients who'd suffered ischemic strokes. The researchers found that all three approaches worked, but that "the combination therapy yielded the most remarkable result, i.e., plasma total homocysteine was reduced by 38.5 percent."[12] A similar British study found a 23 percent decrease in homocysteine levels after six weeks of treatment with folic acid and B_{12}.[13] Evidence indicates that equally impressive results can be achieved by the majority of people who stick with the vitamin regimen.

Does it help to lower high homocysteine levels?

The short answer is: almost certainly yes. Because the medical community's interest in homocysteine's role in cardiovascular disease is new, doctors are still collecting information about how effective a tool homocysteine-lowering therapy will be. Some studies show no effects of lowering homocysteine levels, but data from other studies indicate that the treatment can dramatically lower the risk of death or debility. Among the findings are the following:

- Swiss researchers offered homocysteine-lowering therapy to half of a group of 553 patients who'd undergone angioplasty to correct coronary artery stenosis (narrowing of the arteries). After one year, the researchers reported, the incidence of "major adverse events"—deaths, nonfatal heart attacks, or the need for repeat angioplasty—was one-third lower in the treatment group.[17]
- In a separate six-month double-blind study (a study in which neither the doctor nor the patient knows which treatment is being given), the same Swiss research group administered folic acid, B_{12} and B_6 (a combination they call "folate treatment"), or a placebo, to 205 patients who'd undergone successful coronary artery angioplasty. They reported that the rate of restenosis—that is, re-narrowing of the arteries after

the angioplasty opened them—was significantly lower in the treatment group than in the placebo group (19.6 percent vs. 37.6 percent), and that this group had less than half the need for a repeated procedure on the targeted lesion. The researchers concluded, "This inexpensive treatment, which has minimal side effects, should be considered as adjunctive therapy for patients undergoing coronary angioplasty."[18]**

- Irish researchers studied patients with a genetic disease called homocystinuria, which causes extremely high levels of homocysteine. Normally, half of people with this disease suffer a heart attack or other "vascular event" by the time they're thirty years old. The researchers placed 158 patients on homocysteine-lowering therapy and report that by the time the patients reached an average age of forty-two, twelve patients had collectively experienced seventeen episodes of pulmonary embolism, heart attack, deep vein thrombosis, or other serious vascular problems. "Without treatment," the researchers noted, "112 vascular events would have been expected."[19] In a similar study, Australian researchers reported a 90 percent reduction in cardiovascular events in people with homocystinuria who received homocysteine-lowering therapy.[20]

- Researchers in the United Kingdom and Norway evaluated eighty-nine men, ranging in age from thirty-nine to sixty-seven, with existing coronary artery disease, to determine if oral B vitamins would have an effect on the health of their

---

**A more recent study (Lange, et al., *New England Journal of Medicine*, 2004), which concluded that B vitamin supplementation was ineffective in preventing restenosis, is misleading because the researchers actually found that patients with elevated homocysteine levels—the primary group for which the therapy would be expected to be effective—indeed did show a decreased level of restenosis. So did women (who are at higher risk than men for pernicious anemia) and diabetics (who are at heightened risk for undiagnosed B$_{12}$ deficiency because many are on the B$_{12}$-lowering drug metformin—and because people with Type 1 diabetes are at elevated risk for other autoimmune disorders, such as pernicious anemia). Thus, in the three groups most likely to have high homocysteine and/or low B12 levels, B vitamin therapy did indeed reduce the rate of restenosis—even though the amount of B$_{12}$ used in this study was inadequate. These findings clearly point out the need to screen patients to determine their individual needs and develop logical treatment plans.

Why the Thirty-Year Wait?

Cardiovascular disease is the nation's leading killer, claiming nearly one million lives each year—40 percent of all deaths. More than 2,600 Americans die of cardiovascular disease each day, or one every 33 seconds.[14] Thus, it's amazing that the discovery of the homocysteine/cardiovascular disease link, more than three decades ago, didn't immediately result in a flurry of research and treatment efforts.

Why the gap between discovery and implementation? The answer involves politics, greed, and ignorance.

In the 1960s, Dr. Kilmer McCully, a pathologist at Harvard Medical School, was studying a group of children who'd suffered strokes or blood clots—problems we associate with adults. These children, it turned out, had inborn errors of metabolism that led to extremely high homocysteine levels, which, in turn, put the children at high risk for "adult" cardiovascular problems.

As Dr. McCully studied these children, he began to wonder: Is this same substance, homocysteine, responsible for premature strokes and atherosclerosis in adults, as well? Do adults who suffer heart attacks at forty or strokes at fifty—decades before these problems arise in less susceptible people—have some form of inherited metabolic error, much like children who suffer strokes or develop atherosclerosis? Eventually, his data led McCully to conclude that adults whose homocysteine levels climbed for a variety of reasons (poor diet, malabsorption, veganism, gastrointestinal surgeries, etc.), or those whose genetic makeup left them vulnerable to deficiencies of folic acid, vitamin B_{12}, or vitamin B_6, could be at drastically increased risk for cardiovascular disease. He concluded, further, that simple vitamin therapy could spare many of these people from the ravages of heart attacks, strokes, and blood clots.

McCully announced his conclusions to the medical world in 1969. At the time, however, doctors were firmly proclaiming that another substance, cholesterol, was the key risk factor for cardiovascular disease—and that's where the research money, and the drug company dollars, were going. When Mc-Cully argued that cholesterol was not the main culprit in heart disease, he was vilified. "My laboratory was removed from the department to another part of the hospital," McCully recalls. "It was made clear to me that I should look elsewhere for support." He left Harvard and his research was swept under the rug, although he quietly continued his crusade to make the world aware of the homocysteine/cardiovascular disease link.

Now, more than thirty years later, researchers around the world are proving this link, and McCully's old colleagues are admitting that he was far ahead of his time. "There is a tremendous avalanche of publications," says McCully. "Now about twenty to thirty publications per month are being published. One estimate I saw is there are now over 1,500 publications on homocysteine and vascular heart disease."[15]

Notes the *Journal of Longevity*, "Dr. McCully's research has been a turning point in health science. If he hadn't been so persistent in the face of criticism by his peers, this entire facet of cardiovascular health—the influence of homocysteine—might have remained hidden and many instances of circulatory problems might have remained mysteries."[16]

arteries. After eight weeks of treatment with folic acid and vitamin B$_{12}$, the subjects' plasma homocysteine levels dropped significantly compared to levels in similar men taking a placebo. In addition, the arteries of men taking the vitamins dilated more efficiently in response to blood flow demands. These findings, the researchers concluded, "support the view that lowering homocysteine, through B vitamin supplementation, may reduce cardiovascular risk."[21]

These reports are exciting, because they indicate that homocysteine-reducing vitamin therapy—an inexpensive, simple, and safe treatment—may significantly reduce the rate of cardiovascular disease. What's more, these studies used low-dose oral B$_{12}$, which is less effective than injected B$_{12}$, or high-dose oral B$_{12}$, in patients with existing deficiencies.

It will take years, of course, for the medical community to clarify the role of homocysteine in causing heart attacks, strokes, and other types of vascular disease. Unfortunately most current studies neglect to include MMA testing of subjects, which must be a part of future studies in order for researchers to fully understand how B_{12} factors into this equation. Given the fact that folic acid, vitamin B_{12}, and vitamin B_6 are virtually risk-free treatments, however, people who discover that their homocysteine levels are high shouldn't take any chances.

"I have always had a very personal interest in heart disease," physician Tedd Mitchell wrote in an article for USA Today*'s weekend magazine.[22] "My grandfather died in his 50s of a massive heart attack. And my father had a quadruple bypass in his 50s. This definitely gives me a 'positive' family history of coronary artery disease."*

Mitchell once wondered why his relatives, who had no apparent risk factors—they were nonsmokers, with no high blood pressure, diabetes, high cholesterol, or obesity—were targets for cardiovascular disease at an early age. Then he read about homocysteine, and he decided to have his own level checked. "Lo and behold," he says, "it was significantly elevated." As a result of the studies he's read, he's altered his life-style: Every day, he takes supplements of folic acid, vitamin B_{12}, and vitamin B_6. "I'm happy to report," he adds, "my homocysteine level is now normal."

While many treatments for cardiovascular disease involve potentially dangerous drugs or surgeries, this is one case in which the expected incidence of significant adverse effects is zero. Moreover, while the field of cardiovascular medicine is rife with controversy, this is one instance in which mainstream and holistic doctors are in total agreement about the choice of treatment. To demonstrate just how universal the recommended treatment protocol is, the website of a major drug company explains, "Homocysteine can be easily controlled by providing your body with folic acid, vitamin B_6, and vitamin B_{12} at amounts exceeding the recommended daily allowances."[23] It's difficult to find many examples of major drug companies telling you to take vitamins!

Although we don't yet know who will benefit and to what degree, homocysteine-lowering therapy may prove to be one of the most powerful and simple preventative measures we can implement for people at risk for cardiovascular disease. While we currently tell patients, "Stop smoking, exercise, lose weight, and lower your cholesterol," a quarter of heart attack victims have none of these risk factors.[24] Similarly, thousands of people each year suffer at early ages from strokes, blood clots, or related problems, even though they're seemingly in excellent health. Many of these people carry very common gene variants that can cause their homocysteine to rise to dangerous levels. For these people in particular, early and accurate testing for high homocysteine and low B$_{12}$ levels might mean the difference between dying young and leading a long, healthy life.

The twenty-one-year-old woman[25] who came to the emergency department of a Canadian hospital suffered from a deadly problem that a young woman shouldn't have: a blood clot lodged in a vein within her kidney. It's a problem that's rare even in older adults, and usually occurs in people who've had kidney transplants or suffered a blow to the abdomen.

More than Just a Vascular Risk

In this chapter, we've focused on homocysteine's deleterious effects on your heart and blood vessels. However, high homocysteine can put you at risk for other serious or even fatal medical problems as well. Elevated homocysteine levels are now linked to:

- cognitive impairment (difficulty thinking)
- dementia
- Alzheimer's disease
- depression
- fetal neural tube defects (linked to high maternal homocysteine levels)

In addition, preliminary evidence suggests an association between high homocysteine levels and:

- inflammatory bowel disease
- osteoporosis
- age-related presbyopia *(farsightedness)*
- complications in both type 1 and type 2 diabetes.[30]

However, the young patient had two risk factors for vascular disease. First, she'd recently started taking oral contraceptives, which slightly increase the risk of developing blood clots. And second, she had very high levels of homocysteine, along with a low serum B_{12} level indicative of a deficiency. Further investigation also revealed that she carried two copies of a particular variant of the MTHFR (methylene tetrahydrofolate reductase) gene that is linked to elevated homocysteine levels in as much as 10 percent of the population.

The doctors told the woman to stop taking her birth control pills, gave her drug treatments to dissolve the clot, and started her on oral folic acid, oral B_{12}, and B_{12} injections. Her homocysteine levels dropped markedly over time, almost assuredly reducing her risk of a future clot dramatically.***

If early testing for high homocysteine ever becomes commonplace, it's possible that such life-threatening vascular events in young people will become far more rare. That's because we may be able to identify tens of thousands of people who can be treated with vitamins at a very early age, before they ever begin to develop the blood vessel lesions that can cause premature heart attacks, blood clots, or strokes.

High homocysteine and pregnancy: risks to both mother and child

We've talked about the risks of high homocysteine to the adult heart, but it can also damage an unborn child. In addition, it can contribute to the development of a very common and a potentially fatal cardiovascular complication in pregnant women.

It's well established that high levels of homocysteine in pregnant women are linked to an increased risk of neural tube defects (see Chapter 6). That's why doctors give pregnant women supplemental folic acid, and why they should give them supplemental vitamin B_{12} as well.

*** Her levels never became completely normal, a problem that her doctors attribute to noncompliance with the folic acid regimen, but which could also stem from the fact that she was switched from injected B_{12} to very low levels of oral B_{12}. In our opinion, given the woman's genetic vulnerability, her original documented B_{12} deficiency, and her high risk of future blood clots, she should have remained on injected B_{12} for life. Six months after treatment, her serum B_{12} was only 255 mcg/dl, indicating a need for either injections or possibly high-dose oral B_{12}. She may have pernicious anemia or some other malabsorption problem that prevents her body from absorbing vitamin B_{12} normally.

In addition, high maternal homocysteine levels are a strong risk factor for preeclampsia, a potentially fatal pregnancy complication characterized by high blood pressure, swelling of the hands and face, and protein in the urine. A recent study, using blood samples taken early in pregnancy, compared fifty-six women who later developed severe preeclampsia to matched control group members who did not develop this complication. The samples from the women who later suffered from preeclampsia contained significantly higher homocysteine levels than samples from problem-free women, with those in the highest 25 percent having an almost three times greater risk of developing preeclampsia than other subjects.[26]

Homocysteine and kidney disease

One group of people who nearly always develop dangerously high homocysteine levels are individuals in end-stage renal disease (ESRD). These people's kidneys no longer function, and they are significantly debilitated, but with dialysis treatment they can live relatively normal lives for years. Their high homocysteine, however, puts them at vastly increased risk for strokes, heart attacks, and other vascular problems.

For the most part, doctors trying to lower the homocysteine levels of patients on dialysis resort to high doses of folic acid. This is because dietary folate is the strongest predictor of plasma homocysteine levels in patients with ESRD. But, as we've noted, folic acid can't lower homocysteine in the absence of sufficient vitamin B$_{12}$.

It's not surprising, therefore, that folate supplementation of patients with ESRD rarely reduces homocysteine to normal levels. To see if adding vitamin B$_{12}$ to the treatment regimen would increase its effectiveness, doctors recently performed a prospective trial involving twenty-four dialysis patients with normal or higher-than-normal folate and B$_{12}$ levels. The patients received either standard therapy (folic acid, vitamin B$_6$, and a small dose of oral B$_{12}$) or standard therapy augmented with injected B$_{12}$.

The researchers found that the injected B$_{12}$ reduced plasma homocysteine levels by an average of 32 percent, even though the patients initially appeared to have adequate B$_{12}$ stores. "Patients with higher baseline plasma homocysteine concentrations," they add, "had the greatest response." They conclude, "Patients with considerable persisting hyperhomocysteinemia despite high-dose folic acid therapy are likely to respond to the addition of hydroxocobalamin [B_{12}], irrespective of their serum vitamin B_{12} concentrations."[27]

In a similar study in Japan, twenty-one hemodialysis patients were randomly assigned to receive folic acid supplements, vitamin B_{12} injections plus folic acid, or a combination of folic acid, vitamin B_6, and injected vitamin B_{12}. At the end of the three-week study, the researchers reported, "Treatment resulted in normalization of fasting homocysteine levels in all 14 patients treated by the combined administration of methylcobalamin (B_{12}) and supplementation of folic acid, regardless of whether there was supplementation of vitamin B_6." They add, "The benefit of methylcobalamin administration on lowering plasma homocysteine levels in hemodialysis patients was remarkable."[28]

There is evidence, too, that homocysteine—in addition to its role in damaging blood vessels—acts, through an entirely different mechanism, as a potent uremic toxin that disrupts normal cellular function.[29] These findings should prompt doctors who treat patients with kidney problems to monitor homocysteine and MMA**** levels, and to provide oral folic acid and injected B_{12} at the first sign of a problem. In our opinion, all dialysis patients should receive B_{12} injections.

Alessandra Perna, M.D. and colleagues point out that chronic renal failure patients "have a high mortality rate, attributable mainly to cardiovascular disease: 9 percent per year, which is 30 times the risk in the general population, and even after age adjustment, cardiovascular disease mortality remains 10 to 20 times higher." It is imperative, for the sake of renal disease sufferers and their families, that we study the likely role that homocysteine plays in this astronomical incidence of heart and blood vessel disease, and investigate as well the role that injected B_{12} can potentially play in helping to reduce these patients' cardiovascular risk.

The relationship between kidney disease and high homocysteine, by the way, raises other interesting questions that should be investigated by researchers. One is the "chicken and egg" type of question: Which comes first, kidney disease or the high homocysteine levels seen in dialysis patients? Elevated homocysteine damages the lining of veins and arteries throughout the body, including those in the kidneys. What per-

---

**** In patients with kidney failure, urine MMA testing needs to be done, rather than serum MMA. Serum MMA can give falsely high values in patients with renal insufficiency, or in those who've experienced significant blood loss or dehydration.

centage of patients genetically prone to high homocysteine levels end up in renal failure because excess homocysteine has been scarring and injuring their kidneys for years? Doctors expect to see high homocysteine levels in patients with kidney failure, but never contemplate the probability that in many cases, elevated homocysteine might be a culprit rather than merely a side effect.

The bottom line: If you're at risk, get tested

It's clear to us, given the evidence that high homocysteine is a powerful risk factor for vascular disease in both young and old people, that screening should become commonplace for people at risk for cardiovascular problems. We believe that homocysteine testing should also become routine for senior citizens, pregnant women, and people with the following risk factors:

- Type I or Type II diabetes
- extended use of medications that can raise homocysteine levels, including lipid-lowering drugs, metformin, levodopa, certain anticonvulsants, and possibly androgens
- renal disease
- autoimmune disease
- thyroid disease
- any of the risk factors we've outlined for B$_{12}$ deficiency

If you're overweight or have hyperlipidemia, don't let your doctor forgo homocysteine testing on the basis that "we already know the reasons for your cardiovascular troubles." Some doctors assume that obesity and high blood lipids are adequate explanations for cardiovascular problems, but the presence of these risk factors doesn't rule out the possibility of others.

Patients with high homocysteine levels should be evaluated for underlying B$_{12}$ deficiency, and should be treated with standard doses of folic acid and vitamin B$_6$, and high-dose B$_{12}$. Even people in the upper range of what's considered normal should be started on homocysteine-lowering therapy, because levels only 12 percent above the highest normal level are linked to a threefold increase in the risk of heart attack.[31] There's no downside to treatment, because the vitamins are completely harmless, and they cost only a few dollars out-of-pocket.

It's important, if your doctor puts you on homocysteine-lowering therapy, to be aware that folic acid therapy alone—a treatment that many doctors recommend—is insufficient to treat high homocysteine in some cases. As we've explained, folic acid and B_{12} work hand-in-hand to lower homocysteine, and all the folic acid in the world won't do you a bit of good if there isn't a plentiful supply of B_{12} in your system to help that folic acid do its job.

Jean, a fifty-seven-year-old insurance agent, exercised regularly, avoided cigarettes, ate a diet high in folic acid, and took folate supplements, in order to keep her cardiovascular system healthy—but, as she eventually learned, it wasn't enough.

Because Jean was experiencing some symptoms of B_{12} deficiency that hadn't been noticed by her family physician or her other doctors, we ordered several tests for low B_{12}. In addition, Jean's homocysteine level was measured. All of her tests (B_{12}, MMA, homocysteine, gastrin, and parietal cell antibody) came back grossly abnormal.

As it turned out, Jean had autoimmune pernicious anemia. Even though she took folic acid supplements and ate a diet rich in this nutrient, her homocysteine level was high, because she had a B_{12} deficiency. Her complete blood count was normal because her blood cells could use excess folic acid instead of B_{12}. (This is why folic acid supplements can mask B_{12} deficiency.)

While folic acid made Jean's complete blood count appear normal, and fooled her initial doctors into missing her true diagnosis, her cells couldn't use folic acid to convert homocysteine to methionine—a process that requires B_{12}. That's why her homocysteine levels soared, putting her at risk for cardiovascular disease and other medical problems.

If you undergo homocysteine-lowering therapy, insist that your doctor first obtain a baseline B_{12} and urinary MMA. As we've noted, folic acid therapy corrects the anemia and enlarged blood cells that doctors generally look for when checking for B_{12} deficiency, but does nothing to stop the neurological damage caused by depleted B_{12} stores. Thus, if you're significantly deficient and your B_{12} levels aren't checked first, folic acid therapy can mask the symptoms of your B_{12} deficiency and allow its devastating neurological consequences—including neuropathy, dementia, and mental illness—to proceed to the point at which they become irreversible. In addition, you may fail to lower your homocysteine to healthy levels, thus placing yourself at continued risk for vascular disease.

The following statement, by hematologist A. C. Anthony, is typical of the warnings given in hematology textbooks: "Be certain B$_{12}$ deficiency does not exist when administering folic acid.... Failure to recognize [B$_{12}$] deficiency as the etiology [origin] of neurologic disease and treatment of [B$_{12}$] deficiency with folate... represent significant extremes of deviation from the dictum *primum non nocere* [first, do no harm]."[32]

Equally important, urinary MMA and B$_{12}$ testing will allow your doctor to tailor your homocysteine-lowering program to your individual needs. In some cases, high-dose oral B$_{12}$ supplements will be sufficient. In others, injected B$_{12}$ will be necessary. Your doctor can't merely guess how much B$_{12}$ is enough for you, or rely on products marketed as homocysteine-lowering medications. (For example, Folgard, an oral vitamin supplement designed to reduce homocysteine, contains 800 micrograms of folic acid, 10 milligrams of vitamin B$_6$, and 115 micrograms of vitamin B$_{12}$. That's fine for people with healthy B$_{12}$ levels and none of the malabsorption problems we outlined earlier. However, for a vitamin B$_{12}$-deficient individual, the oral dosage of B$_{12}$ needs to be 1,000 to 2,000 micrograms daily—and, as we've noted, some patients respond better with injections.) With the health of your vascular system at stake, it's worth the extra effort to make sure you're getting the most effective treatment possible.

Rethinking Fortified Cereals

The United States fortifies many foods with folic acid, and Great Britain is working on implementing a similar plan. Given the link between homocysteine and heart disease, both countries should consider fortifying foods with vitamin B$_{12}$ as well. British researchers recently conducted a study in which fifty-three healthy adults received increasing doses of folic acid over a six-month period. At the beginning of the study, the subjects' levels of homocysteine dropped in response to this nutrient. But as the folic acid dosage increased, homocysteine levels dropped less in response to this vitamin and more in response to vitamin B$_{12}$.

This finding, the researchers say, "suggests that a fortification policy based on folic acid and vitamin B$_{12}$, rather than folic acid alone, is likely to be much more effective at lowering... homocysteine concentrations, with potential benefits for reduction of risk of vascular disease."[33]

Notes

1. Abbott Laboratories, http://www.abbott.com.my/t_healthv_main.html
2. "Hot health tips," USC Care Medical Group, http://www.usc.edu/health/uscp/hhtsuddenheart.html.
3. Nygard, O., Nordrehaug, J. E., Refsum, H., Ueland, P. M., Farstad, M., and Vollset, S. E. Plasma homocysteine levels and mortality in patients with coronary artery disease. *New England Journal of Medicine* 1997, 337:230–6.
4. O'Callaghan, P. and Graham, I. Update on homocysteine. *Heartwise* (Irish Heart Foundation), Winter 2000.
5. Booth, G. L., and Wang, E. E. Preventive health care 2000 update: Screening and management of hyperhomocysteinemia for the prevention of coronary artery disease events. The Canadian Task Force on Preventive Health Care. *Canadian Medical Association Journal* 2000, 163(1):21–9.
6. Kark, J. D., Sinnreich, R., Rosenberg, I. H., Jacques, P. F., and Selhub, J. Plasma homocysteine and parental myocardial infarction in young adults in Jerusalem. *Circulation* 2002, 105(23):2725–9.
7. Stampfer, M. J., Malinow, M. R., Willett, W. C., Newcomer, L. M, Upson, B., Ullmann, D., Tishler, P. V., and Hennekens, C. H. *Journal of the American Medical Association* 1992, 268(7):877–81.
8. Nygard, O., Nordrehaug, J. E., Refsum, H., Ueland, P. M., Farstad, M., and Vollset, S. E. Plasma homocysteine levels and mortality in patients with coronary artery disease. *New England Journal of Medicine* 1997, 337:230–6.
9. Stubbs, P. J., Al-Obaidi, M. K., Conroy, R. M., Collinson, P. O., Graham, I. M., and Noble, M. Effect of plasma homocysteine concentration on early and late events in patients with acute coronary syndromes. *Circulation* 2000, 102:605–10.
10. Wald, D. S., Law, M., and Morris, J. K. Homocysteine and cardiovascular disease: Evidence on causality from a meta-analysis. *British Medical Journal* 2002, 325:1202.
11. Kittner, S. J., Giles, W. H., Macko, R. F., Hebel, J. R., Wozniak, M. A., Wityk, R. J., Stolley, P. D., Stern, B. J., Sloan, M. A., Sherwin, R., Price, T. R., McCarter, R. J., Johnson, C. J., Earley, C. J., Buchholz, D. W., and Malinow, M. R. Homocyst(e)ine and risk of cerebral infarction in a biracial population: The stroke prevention in young women study. *Stroke* 1999, 30(8):1554–60; and, "Study links vitamin B deficiency to risk of stroke in younger women." *Doctor's Guide*, August 30, 1999, http://www.docguide.com.
12. Sato, Y., Kaji, M., Kondo, I., Yoshida, H., Satoh, K., and Metoki, N. Hyperhomocysteinemia in Japanese patients with convalescent stage ischemic stroke: Effect of combined therapy with folic acid and mecobalamine. *Journal of the Neurological Sciences* 2002, 202(1–2):65–8.

13. MacMahon, M., Kirkpatrick, C., Cummings, C. E., Clayton, A., Robinson, P. J., Tomiak, R. H., Liu, M., Kush, D., and Tobert, J. *Nutrition, Metabolism, and Cardiovascular Diseases* 2000, 10(4):195–203.

14. Statistics are from the American Heart Association, *2002 Heart and Stroke Statistical Update.*

15. Quotes are from Dr. McCully's discussion with Richard Passwater, Ph.D., at NutritionFocus.com, http.//www.nutritionfocus.com/nutrition_library/ homocysteine.html, and from Bucco, Gloria, "Kilmer McCully, M.D., connects homocysteine and heart disease," *Nutrition Science News*, July 1999.

16. Yutsis, P. Homocysteine or cholesterol: Which is more deadly? *Journal of Longevity*, http://www.journaloflongevity.com/JOLWeb/Archives/86/ deadly.html.

17. Schnyder, G., Roffi, M., Flammer, Y., Pin, R., and Hess, O. M. Effect of homocysteine-lowering therapy with folic acid, vitamin B(12), and vitamin B(6) on clinical outcome after percutaneous coronary intervention. The Swiss Heart Study: a randomized controlled trial. *Journal of the American Medical Association* 2002, 288(8):973–9.

18. Schnyder, G., Roffi, M., Pin, R., Flammer, Y., Lange, H., Eberli, F. R., Meier, B., Turi, Z. G., and Hess, O. M. Decreased rate of coronary restenosis after lowering of plasma homocysteine levels. *New England Journal of Medicine* 2001, 345(22):1593–600.

19. Yap, S., Boers, G. H., Wilcken, B., Wilcken, D. E., Brenton, D. P., Lee, P. J., Walter, J. H., Howard, P. M., and Naughten, E. R. Vascular outcome in patients with homocystinuria due to cystathionine beta-synthase deficiency treated chronically: a multicenter observational study. *Arteriosclerosis, Thrombosis, and Vascular Biology* 2001, 21(12):2080–5.

20. Ueland, P. M., Refsum, H., Beresford, S. A. A., and Vollset, S. E. The controversy over homocysteine and cardiovascular risk. *American Journal of Clinical Nutrition* 2000, 72:324–32.

21. Chambers, J. C., Ueland, P. M., Obeid, O. A., Wrigley, J., Refsum, H., and Kooner. J. S. Improved vascular endothelial function after oral B vitamins. An effect mediated through reduced concentrations of free plasma homocysteine. *Circulation* 2000, 102:2479–83.

22. Mitchell, Tedd. At the heart of a family mystery. USAweekend.com, February 25, 2001.

23. http://www.abbott.com.my/t_healthv_main.html

24. http://www.abbott.com.my/t_healthv_main.html

25. This woman's case appears in Chan, H. H. W., Douketis, J. D., and Nowaczyk, M. J. M. Acute renal vein thrombosis, oral contraceptive use, and hyperhomocysteinemia. *Mayo Clinic Proceedings* 2001, 76:212–214.

26. Cotter, A. M., Molloy, A. M., Scott, J. M., and Daly, S. F. Elevated plasma homocysteine in early pregnancy: a risk factor for the development of severe preeclampsia. *American Journal of Obstetrics and Gynecology* 2001, 185(4):781–5.

27. Elian, K. M., and Hoffer, L. J. Hydroxocobalamin reduces hyperhomocys-teinemia in end-stage renal disease. *Metabolism* 2002, 51(7):881–6.

28. Koyama, K., Usami, T., Takeuchi, O., Morozumi, K., and Kimura, G. Efficacy of methylcobalamin on lowering total homocysteine plasma concentrations in haemodialysis patients receiving high-dose folic acid supplementation. *Nephrology, Dialysis, Transplantation* 2002, 17(5):916–22.

29. Perna, A. F., Castaldo, P., Ingross, D., and De Santo, N. Homocysteine, a new cardiovascular risk factor, is also a powerful uremic toxin. *Journal of Nephrology* 1999, 12:230–40.

30. References for information in this chart include: Herrmann, W. and Knapp, J-P. Hyperhomocysteinemia: A new risk factor for degenerative diseases. *Clinical Laboratory* 2002, 48:471–81; Krumdieck, C. L. and Prince, C. W. Mechanisms of homocysteine toxicity on connective tissues: Implications for the morbidity of aging. *Journal of Nutrition* 2000, 130(2S Suppl):365S–368S; Romagnuolo, J., Fedorak, R. N., Dias, V. C., Bamforth, F., and Teltscher, M. Hyperhomocysteinemia and inflammatory bowel disease: Prevalence and predictors in a cross-sectional study. *American Journal of Gastroenterology* 2001, 96(7):2143–9; Kark, J. D., Selhub, J., Bostom, A., Adler, B., and Rosenberg, I. H. Plasma homocys-teine and all-cause mortality in diabetes. *The Lancet* 1999, 353:1936–7; and Agullo-Ortuno, M. T., Albaladejo, M. D., Parra, S., Rodriguez-Manotas, M., Fenollar, M., Ruiz-Espejo, F., Tebar, J., and Martinez, P. Plasmatic homocysteine concentration and its relationship with complica-tions associated to diabetes mellitus. *Clinica Chimica Acta* 2002, 326(1–2):105–12.

31. Chambers, J. C., Ueland, P. M., Obeid, O. A., Wrigley, J., Refsum, H., and Kooner, J. S. Improved vascular endothelial function after oral B vita-mins: An effect mediated through reduced concentrations of free plasma homocysteine. *Circulation* 2000, 102:2479–83.

32. Antony, A. C. Megaloblastic anemias. In R. Hoffman, et al., *Hematology: Basic Principles and Practice*, 3rd edition, 2000, Philadelphia: Churchill Livingstone.

33. Quinlivan, E. P., McPartlin, J., McNulty, H., Ward, M., Strain, J. J, Weir, D. G., and Scott, J. M. Importance of both folic acid and vitamin B_{12} in reduction of risk of vascular disease. *Lancet* 2002, 359(9302):227–8.

6

Lost Children: When B_{12} Deficiency Causes Developmental Disabilities or Learning Problems

"My baby became symptomatic, not me. The result was irreversible brain damage in my breast-fed child." —A B_{12}-deficient mother

If you're a parent, protecting your child from danger is your biggest concern. But no matter how cautious you are, there's one danger that you may not recognize: the risk that your child may suffer, both physically and mentally, from a B_{12} deficiency. Low B_{12} levels severely damage the brains of hundreds of children each year, and new research shows that subclinical mental deficits may occur in tens of thousands more.

In some cases, children suffer irreversible brain damage because they have inborn defects of B_{12} metabolism that doctors fail to identify. In other cases, environmental factors—primarily diet—are to blame. Unfortunately, doctors know far too little about either inborn or acquired B_{12} problems. Parents, as well, often aren't aware that breast-feeding their babies during infancy, and feeding them healthy meals when they're older, won't guarantee they'll be safe. In fact, ironically, it's often the most health-conscious mothers who put their children at greatest risk.

Lisa smiled, sat up, and said "Mama" and "Dada" right on schedule, but when she turned eight months old, something went terribly wrong.

She stopped talking. She couldn't stand up or grasp her toys. She stopped responding with smiles and coos to the people around her. Even-

tually, she couldn't even sit up without help. Her arms writhed in a snake-like way, an indication of brain damage. Her eyes fixed on people, but didn't follow them when they moved. She was frail and short, and her head was abnormally small for her age.

Lisa's doctors must have weighed many different diagnoses as she regressed in front of their eyes: autism, Rett syndrome, Tay-Sachs' disease, or a tumor or infection. But they missed an easy call, and in doing so, they nearly robbed her of the chance to lead a normal life.

When Lisa was fourteen months old, her parents took her to a new doctor who took note of the fact that she'd been breast-fed by a vegetarian mother who ate few of the animal products that contain B$_{12}$. A test of the mother's B$_{12}$ level came back low but in the normal range, but Lisa's levels were depleted. Immediate treatment with B$_{12}$ led to rapid improvement in Lisa's symptoms, and she quickly grew taller and put on weight. Nine years later, the doctor reported, she was completely normal.[1]

Lisa owes her functioning brain and body to this doctor, who spotted her B$_{12}$ deficiency six months after her symptoms occurred—probably at almost the last minute that treatment could completely reverse her neurologic damage. If he'd missed the diagnosis, as her previous doctors had, Lisa would most likely be mentally retarded and wheelchair-bound for the rest of her life.

In adults, B$_{12}$ deficiency is often insidious, taking its toll over years or even decades. In children, however, a severe deficiency can strike with terrifying swiftness. Within months, a happy, babbling, cooing, crawling infant can be reduced to a child who appears half-conscious and can barely lift its head. Babies and toddlers affected by severe B$_{12}$ deficiency begin to lose their speech and social skills, and they become apathetic and irritable. They often refuse to eat, and they regress to the point where they can no longer sit, crawl, stand, or walk. Their heads and bodies grow too slowly, and they fail to gain weight, becoming thin and weak. Brain scans frequently show atrophy of the cerebral cortex.

If caught in time, B$_{12}$ deficiency can be corrected quickly, and affected infants and toddlers can regain all of their skills and receive a good prognosis for a full recovery. Sadly, however, many cases aren't diagnosed until children become permanently learning-disabled or even mentally retarded. And many cases, involving much milder and harder-to-detect symptoms, are never diagnosed at all.

Some children are genetically destined to develop B$_{12}$ deficiency, a problem we'll discuss later in this chapter and more extensively in Chapter 12. Thousands of other children have borderline or even dangerously low B$_{12}$ levels because of what they eat (or, more correctly, what they *don't* eat). And many others have a "second-hand" deficiency, starting in their earliest days of life, because their mothers had deficient levels of B$_{12}$ during pregnancy or while breast-feeding.

When mothers are deficient in B$_{12}$, the damage to their babies starts in the womb. You've probably heard of neural tube defects (NTDs), which are very common, severe birth defects occurring when the brain or spinal cord fails to form correctly. Low levels of folic acid increase the risk for NTDs, which is why doctors now ensure that their pregnant patients get plenty of this vitamin. However, research also strongly implicates low B$_{12}$ levels as a factor in NTDs[2]—which isn't surprising, since folic acid and B$_{12}$ work hand in hand. (You'll remember from earlier chapters that for the body to use folic acid, vitamin B$_{12}$ must be present.) In addition, studies show that children of severely B$_{12}$-deficient mothers exhibit abnormal behavior stemming from dysfunction of the basal ganglia (a part of the brain that helps control movement and emotional regulation) and pyramidal tracts (pathways linking the motor cortex to the spinal cord).[3] Studies of animals also link B$_{12}$ deficiency to an increased risk of stillbirth and infant death, as well as to low birth weight in newborns.[4]

Even women with adequate stores of B$_{12}$ can damage their unborn babies' brains if they fail to take in enough B$_{12}$ in their diet. Because only newly-absorbed vitamin B$_{12}$ readily crosses the placenta, the vitamin B$_{12}$ stockpiled by the mother's body is largely ineffective in protecting the health of the fetus.[5]

Worse, the danger of second-hand B$_{12}$ deficiency doesn't end the day a baby is born. Mothers with depleted B$_{12}$ stores, who exclusively breast-feed their babies, unknowingly put them at great risk for developmental disability or even death. This is a common cause of B$_{12}$ problems in infants; one study, for instance, found that half of a group of six infants diagnosed with crippling B$_{12}$ deficiency became ill after being nursed by vegetarian mothers. (The other half were born to mothers with undiagnosed pernicious anemia [an autoimmune disease].)[6]

Vegetarian and vegan mothers are devastated and feel tremendous guilt when their children suffer harm due to B$_{12}$ deficiency, but in reality most of these tragedies are the fault of doctors who fail to screen pregnant and nursing mothers for this deficiency—and who then often misdiagnose these women's children as mentally retarded or autistic, rather than considering B$_{12}$ deficiency, when the infants lose their speech, social skills, and motor skills. Because B$_{12}$ occurs naturally only in animal products, a vegan diet, which excludes eggs and dairy products as well as meat and fish, provides virtually no natural B$_{12}$. A vegetarian diet, while it can include eggs and cheese, may provide too little B$_{12}$, especially if a mother has any of the risk factors that make her vulnerable to B$_{12}$ deficiency (see Chapter 1). A macrobiotic diet, which excludes most animal protein with the exception of fish, also can lead to B$_{12}$ depletion. And even vegan, vegetarian, or macrobiotic-diet mothers who take B$_{12}$ supplements can easily become deficient, if they take too low a dose—a common occurrence—or if they have trouble absorbing the vitamin.

Another problem occurs when mothers on no-animal-protein diets take ineffective supplements. Studies show that vegetarian formulations of B$_{12}$ supplements don't always dissolve well, meaning that even a correct dosage of the vitamin can pass through the gastrointestinal tract largely undigested.[7] In addition, many vegans supplement their diets with spirulina (an algae), tempeh (fermented soy), or nori (a seaweed) in the belief that these plant foods contain vitamin B$_{12}$—a widely accepted idea based on laboratory tests that showed significant amounts of the vitamin in these plants. Newer research, however, shows that the tests are primarily detecting "pseudo-vitamin B$_{12}$" analogues that may actually block the uptake of real B$_{12}$.[8]

Pseudo-B$_{12}$ also shows up as real B$_{12}$ in blood tests, meaning that spirulina-consuming vegetarians with "normal" B$_{12}$ levels may actually be severely deficient. Nutritionist Stephen Byrnes recently wrote, "In my own practice, I recently saved two vegans from death from anemia by convincing them to eat generous amounts of dairy products. Both of [them] thought their B$_{12}$ needs were being met by tempeh and spirulina. They weren't."[9]

Vegetarian and vegan mothers also are the most likely to breastfeed for long periods of time, which puts nursing children at high risk of B$_{12}$ deficiency if the mothers don't supplement their diets correctly. Children can be severely crippled by B$_{12}$ deficiency even if their breast-feeding vegan mothers have normal B$_{12}$ levels, because, as in the case of pregnancy, the mother's body will not mobilize existing stores of B$_{12}$ efficiently in order to make up for a dietary deficiency. "Consequently," hematologist Julian Davis and his colleagues say, "even mothers who have only recently become vegans and who have no hematologic or biochemical evidence of vitamin B$_{12}$ deficiency may place their nurslings at risk for this vitamin deficiency."[10] Adding to this risk, babies who are B$_{12}$-deficient often become anorexic and reject solid foods, leading mothers to breast-feed them even longer and further worsen their B$_{12}$ deficiency.

A growing risk

A 1997 Roper Poll estimated that between half a million and two million Americans are practicing vegans, with a far larger number eating vegetarian diets, macrobiotic diets, or other diets very low in animal products. Vegetarian, vegan, and macrobiotic diets are growing in popularity, particularly among young people and particularly among females of child-bearing age. Given the overall healthfulness of vegan/vegetarian diets, this is a good thing—*except* when the people following these otherwise-healthy diets fail to get enough B$_{12}$.

Unfortunately, that's a common occurrence. Among the findings of researchers are the following:

- "Serum vitamin [B$_{12}$] levels are significantly lower in subjects consuming alternative nutrition, with deficiency observed in 24 percent of vegetarians and 78 percent of vegans vs. 0 percent in omnivores."[11]
- "The increased MMA concentration suggested a 25 percent frequency of functional vitamin B$_{12}$ deficiency [in vegetarians]."[12]
- "The prevalence of hyperhomocysteinemia [a strong indicator of B$_{12}$ deficiency, if kidney disease and thyroid disease are not present] was higher in vegetarians (53.3 percent) than in controls (10.3 percent)."[13]
- "Evidence indicates that over 80 percent of those people who have been vegans for two years or more are deficient in cobalamin [B$_{12}$] as determined by a serum cobalamin below 250 pg/ml and/or an elevated level of urinary MMA."[14]

These findings should place gynecologists and pediatricians on alert. As the numbers of vegetarian and vegan women grow, so too, almost inevitably, will the problem of babies suffering from preventable brain and nervous system damage when their mothers are not educated about proper B$_{12}$ supplementation. The solution is simple: Doctors, dietitians, and other health professionals must ensure that women following a vegetarian or vegan diet receive in-depth information about the necessity for B$_{12}$ supplements, accurate information about which supplements work and which don't, and regular tests of their MMA levels during pregnancy and nursing.

None of this is a criticism of meat-free diets, which—because they are low in fat, high in phytochemicals and antioxidants, and generally low in artificial colorings and additives—tend to be very healthful. If they contain plenty of supplemental B$_{12}$, vegan or vegetarian or macrobiotic diets can help the heart and reduce the risk of cancer and diabetes. But without adequate B$_{12}$, the same diets can be a death sentence—not only for adults, but for the children they love.

Other mothers, other risks

While vegan or vegetarian mothers are the most likely to be low in B$_{12}$, even mothers who eat large amounts of meat and other animal products may be B$_{12}$-deficient and not know it. Women at highest risk include those with undiagnosed pernicious anemia, those who've undergone gastrointestinal surgery (including weight-loss surgeries), those with family histories of pernicious anemia, those who eat poorly during pregnancy, and those with autoimmune or malabsorption disorders—but a woman who has none of these risk factors, and appears completely healthy, can still be starving her baby of B$_{12}$.

A recent study, in fact, showed that one third of infants develop elevated MMA levels by six weeks of age, a possible sign of inadequate levels of B$_{12}$. "Notably," the researchers say, "we studied consecutive pregnancies in healthy, well-nourished mothers who consumed an omnivorous, non-vegetarian diet, and even in this population we found biochemical evidence of cobalamin [B$_{12}$] deficiency."[15]

This finding was particularly true for infants who were not firstborns. This indicates, they say, that "the prevalence of impaired cobalamin status in the neonatal period may be underestimated"—a mistake that could lead to thousands of children suffering subtle but permanent neurologic damage.

This is why we believe that at-risk women who are pregnant need to have a urinary MMA test—particularly if they plan to nurse their babies.* Testing is especially important for pregnant teens, who often eat poor diets; a recent study of fifty-eight pregnant adolescents showed that twenty-five had suboptimal serum B$_{12}$ levels.[16]

In addition, any infant with an unexplained developmental disability should be screened immediately for B$_{12}$ deficiency. Babies and toddlers diagnosed quickly are highly likely to make full recoveries, while those who go months or years without a diagnosis are likely to suffer permanent neurological damage and become mentally retarded. The nervous system develops most rapidly during the first two years, and the brain reaches full growth and maturity by age six, so the early months and years are the most critical for detection and correction of B$_{12}$ deficiency.

Jamie developed normally until he became lethargic and irritable at four months of age. When Jamie was eight months old, a doctor noted his small head size, and his inability to sit unsupported or lift his head when placed on his back or tummy. Jamie also moved his limbs in an abnormal, snakelike motion, and his eyes failed to fix on a toy, or follow movements.

Tests showed that Jamie's mother had pernicious anemia and a severely low serum B$_{12}$ level of 128 pg/ml. Unaware of her deficiency, she'd breast-fed Jamie, thinking she was providing him with the best diet possible.

"The child's response to vitamin B$_{12}$ supplements was remarkable," his doctors say, "with an improvement in head growth up to the 90th percentile, disappearance of the [abnormal movements], and improved development." However, follow-up tests five years later showed that the boy suffered from borderline intellectual retardation—a permanent consequence of his early lack of B$_{12}$.[17]

Childhood and adolescence: B$_{12}$ deficiency and learning problems

Every year, several million parents put their children on vegetarian, vegan, or macrobiotic diets. At the same time, millions of adolescents

---

* Serum B$_{12}$ levels in pregnant women have been shown to give false positive test results (low levels in the absence of deficiency), so the urinary MMA is preferred.

choose, either for health reasons or for philosophical reasons, to forgo meat and animal products.

Again, this is a valid decision—*if* these children and teens obtain the right amounts of supplemental B$_{12}$ (as well as adequate levels of iron and other nutrients), and if they have no medical problems that prevent them from absorbing B$_{12}$ properly. Research indicates, however, that a large number of non-meat-eating children aren't getting enough vitamin B$_{12}$ either in their diets or from supplements, and that their brains aren't functioning optimally as a result.

In 1985, Dr. Wija van Staveren and colleagues began following a group of infants being raised on vegan diets. Because these diets contain no animal products, they are extremely low in vitamin B$_{12}$. Testing the children in their early years, the researchers noticed subtle but significant impairments in the psychomotor functioning of the vegan children as compared to those eating meat and dairy products.

Told of these findings, many parents of the vegan children participating in the study chose to switch their children to diets containing milk, eggs, and in some cases meat. On average, the children began eating animal products at around the age of six. When the children reached adolescence, the researchers again compared them to a group of children raised from birth on diets including animal products. Each of the forty-eight formerly-vegan children and the twenty-four control children took a ninety-minute battery of tests that measured their cognitive skills, and the researchers measured their serum B$_{12}$ and MMA levels.

Many of the children raised until age six on vegan diets were still B$_{12}$-deficient, even after years of eating at least some animal proteins. "We found a significant association between cobalamin [B$_{12}$] status and performance on tests measuring fluid intelligence, spatial ability, and short-term memory," Staveren and colleagues say, with the formerly-vegan children scoring lower than the control group members in each case.

The deficit in the early-vegan children's fluid intelligence is particularly troubling, the researchers say, "because it involves reasoning, the capacity to solve complex problems, abstract thinking ability, and the ability to learn. Any defect in this area may have far-reaching consequences for individual functioning."

Most of the children switched from vegan diets had B$_{12}$ intakes close to the Recommended Dietary Allowance at the time of the follow-up study, yet many of them continued to suffer from B$_{12}$ deficiency. "Because these subjects consumed a diet extremely low in cobalamin [B$_{12}$] from birth up to the age of six years," the researchers say, "their cobalamin stores may never have reached an optimal level and moderate intakes may not have been sufficient for obtaining normal serum cobalamin status."[18]**

There are three lessons to be learned from this study. One is that an alarming percentage of people who put their children on vegetarian, vegan, and macrobiotic diets are failing to do the right thing when it comes to B$_{12}$ supplements. Another is that children on these diets need to have their urine MMA status checked regularly, and they need B$_{12}$ injections if high-dose oral supplements aren't keeping their levels of the vitamin high enough. And a third lesson is that if your child becomes B$_{12}$-deficient, simply switching him or her to a diet higher in B$_{12}$ and offering a multivitamin supplement may not be enough. Children with B$_{12}$ deficiency need higher-than-normal amounts of the vitamin in order to replenish their depleted stores, just as adults do, and the standard vitamin formulas that parents typically buy are not up to the job. (For example, Flintstones children's multivitamins—which are similar to most oral vitamin preparations for children—contain only six micrograms of B$_{12}$, compared to the 1,000 micrograms needed daily if oral B$_{12}$ is taken to correct a deficiency.)***

Symptoms: from subtle to severe

Like the children in the study by Dr. van Staveren and colleagues, many B$_{12}$-deficient children have symptoms too subtle to be picked up by most doctors, or even by parents. Their mental symptoms—memory deficits, slight declines in fluid IQ, fatigue, mood changes—may be written off as behavior problems, "growing pains," or even mild learning disabilities. As a consequence, the children may wind up on Ritalin or other drugs rather than receiving a proper diagnosis.

**It's puzzling that although the parents of the children in this study were highly educated, and researchers detected the children's low cobalamin status in infancy, a number of these children's personal physicians apparently did not conduct regular B$_{12}$ testing during childhood, or provide B$_{12}$ injections when needed—the only likely explanation for the children's continuing deficiency. We would consider this to be substandard medical care for children with identified deficiencies.

*** See Chapter 10 for more information.

In some cases, however, the symptoms seen in children and teens are dramatic, resembling those of middle-aged adults or senior citizens with drastic B_{12} depletion. Symptoms can range from muscle weakness and learning problems to paralysis, psychiatric disorders, or even blindness. And as with adults, children can undergo drastic neurological deterioration even when standard blood tests show no signs of B_{12} deficiency anemia.

The first thing fourteen-year-old "F. C." noticed was that his calf hurt when he stood up. The pain grew worse and worse, and soon he began stumbling and falling. Eventually, he needed help walking.

Examining F. C., a physician learned that the boy suffered from fatigue and daytime sleepiness. F. C. was small for his age and thin, weighing only eighty-eight pounds, and his heart beat too slowly. He seemed "flat" emotionally, and he answered the doctor's questions in monosyllables, cooperating momentarily and then becoming withdrawn.

Learning that F. C. was a longtime vegan and a picky eater, the doctor suspected B_{12} deficiency. Tests showed a normal serum B_{12} level, but massively elevated MMA and homocysteine levels, indicating severe B_{12} depletion.

When the doctor gave F. C. B_{12} injections, the boy quickly regained his ability to walk. In addition, when the mental deficits caused by F. C.'s low B_{12} levels disappeared, his aloofness and lack of emotion vanished, and he once again responded normally to his friends and family. F. C.'s MMA and homocysteine levels were normal at follow-up, although he continued to show some neurologic abnormalities eighteen months after diagnosis.[19]

While children eating vegan or vegetarian diets are the most likely to have deficient B_{12} levels, they aren't the only young people prone to develop a deficiency. The same risk factors that apply to adults—any history of gastrointestinal disease (particularly Crohn's disease) or surgery, the presence of any autoimmune disorder (especially thyroid disease), celiac disease or gluten intolerance, the presence of iron deficiency, use of B_{12}-lowering medications, any unexplained neurological or mental symptoms, or any lengthy exposure to nitrous oxide (either during surgery or dental work, or as a drug of abuse)—apply to children and teens, and should lead parents and doctors to suspect possible

B$_{12}$ deficiency. Teens with bulimia or anorexia should also be checked for B$_{12}$ deficiency, because they are prone to subclinical nutritional deficiencies.

Most pediatric cases involving neurological damage due to acquired B$_{12}$ deficiency, however, involve children eating vegan, vegetarian, or macrobiotic diets. Parents who implement such diets can avoid these tragedies by researching the issue of B$_{12}$ supplementation thoroughly, and having their children's urinary MMA levels (and their own, if they are pregnant or nursing women) tested regularly. As Joel Fuhrman, a physician and a practicing vegetarian, says, "It is entirely irresponsible for a health professional not to recommend B$_{12}$ supplementation in some form or frequent monitoring of MMA with blood tests for those who do not consume any animal products in their diets. No controversy exists."[20] This is true for all vegetarians and vegans, and it's particularly true in the case of the youngest and most vulnerable—the babies and children who trust their parents, and their doctors, to protect their health.

Developmental disorders: the B$_{12}$ link

Not all cases of B$_{12}$ deficiency in infancy stem from an inadequate diet. A number of children suffer, instead, from genetic flaws that impair some aspect of the complex process of B$_{12}$ metabolism. In fact, there are ten different inherited defects that are known to impair the pathways of B$_{12}$ metabolism and transport in humans. Seven alter cellular utilization and coenzyme production, and the other three affect absorption and transport. All of these disorders can severely damage a child—especially if they aren't detected early.

Unfortunately, while children undergo testing at birth for phenylketonuria (PKU) and other inborn errors of metabolism, the officials who decide what tests to provide often neglect errors of B$_{12}$ metabolism. Only twelve states and the District of Columbia currently test for homocystinuria, for instance, and none of the fifty states tests for methylmalonic aciduria. Yet either of these two conditions, which often stem from inborn errors of B$_{12}$ metabolism, can be fatal—and even when they aren't, the damage that occurs when they go undetected is incalculable.

In a recent issue of Discover, *physician Mark Cohen describes the frantic phone call he received from a mother one day. The woman's daughter Jennifer, at three and a half years of age, suffered from a developmen-*

tal disability of unknown origin, and doctors tentatively diagnosed her as autistic because she showed little affection, played only by herself, showed no imagination, and did not speak normally.

The day Jennifer's mother called, the little girl had been fine at school. When she came home, however, her mother said, "She sat down to play, and when she stood up, she couldn't walk right, like she was dizzy. And she just doesn't seem to be herself."

She took Jennifer to Dr. Cohen's office, where he spotted troubling signs and symptoms: The toddler lurched when she walked, fell several times, turned her head to the right to look at objects, and used her left but not her right hand.

"I think this little girl has had a stroke," Dr. Cohen said. An MRI, indeed, revealed a stroke caused by a blood clot, and further tests revealed a "sky high" homocysteine level. The diagnosis: homocystinuria, an inborn error of metabolism that often involves a disruption in the B$_{12}$ pathway. When homocystinuria is identified early, treatment will prevent strokes and other damage.****

When Jennifer received treatment for her disorder, she began smiling and interacting, started playing with toys, began learning sign language, and no longer appeared autistic. She has not suffered another stroke since treatment began.

A happy ending? Not really. Jennifer almost assuredly wouldn't have suffered her first stroke, or developed autistic behaviors, if her state tested children at birth or early in life for homocystinuria, just as they test children for PKU and other inborn errors of metabolism. Her disorder also could have been identified early on if any of the specialists who saw Jennifer over the three and a half years of her life had ordered tests for inborn errors of B$_{12}$ metabolism.[21]

In most cases, children with inborn errors of B$_{12}$ metabolism develop severe symptoms within the first few months of life. Sometimes, however, symptoms—typically difficulty in walking, and mental and cog-

---

****B$_{12}$ (hydroxocobalamin) therapy is essential only in specific forms of homocystinuria. Because homocystinuria can also stem from an inborn error in the metabolism of B$_6$ or folic acid, not all children respond to B$_{12}$; some require treatment with folate, vitamin B$_6$, a combination of vitamins, betaine, and/or alterations in the protein or amino acid content of their diet (see Chapter 12).

nitive problems—don't appear until the affected children reach toddler-
hood, childhood, the teen years, or even early adulthood. These late-onset errors of metabolism may not be picked up during newborn screening. Thus, any infants, children, teens, or young adults who develop neurologic symptoms should be tested for inborn errors of B$_{12}$ metabolism.

Such testing rarely occurs, however, because few doctors are familiar with these conditions. Says genetic pediatric researcher Piero Rinaldo,
M.D., "As a matter of fact, you cannot diagnose what you don't know,
and unfortunately a large proportion of cases remain undiagnosed because these disorders are not yet included in mainstream medical practice."[22] This oversight can have fatal medical consequences—and devastating legal consequences as well.

*In 1989, Patricia Stallings rushed her infant son, Ryan, to the emer-
gency department, after he became lethargic, vomited his food, and developed trouble breathing. Lab tests ordered by the hospital's doctors
showed the presence of ethylene glycol (a substance found in antifreeze)
in Ryan's blood. Believing that Stallings had tried to poison Ryan, the
authorities placed him in foster care, allowing Patricia only brief visits,
during which she could hold and feed him. Shortly after one of these
visits, Ryan became desperately ill and was rushed to the hospital, where
he died. Suspecting Stallings of again poisoning her son, police arrested
her. A jury convicted her of first degree murder, and Patricia went to
prison. At the time, she was pregnant with her second son—a child who
would be the key to her freedom.*

*Patricia's second child, David, entered foster care immediately af-
ter his birth. Shortly afterward, he began developing symptoms eerily
similar to Ryan's. David's doctors diagnosed him with methylmalonic
acidemia, an inborn error of B$_{12}$ metabolism, and immediately began
appropriate treatment. Concerned that he might have sent an innocent
woman to prison, the attorney who prosecuted Patricia Stallings consulted with several doctors and finally asked Dr. Piero Rinaldo (the researcher cited earlier in this chapter) to investigate. Dr. Rinaldo conclusively determined that Ryan's symptoms, like his brother's, stemmed from
methylmalonic acidemia. The two labs that analyzed Ryan's blood had
used older gas chromatography techniques that confused one of the substances elevated in Ryan's disorder with ethylene glycol.*

The prosecutor dismissed the charges against Patricia Stallings, but *by then she'd lost a year of her life for the "crime" of having a baby with an inborn error of B$_{12}$ metabolism. Worse yet, Rinaldo says, the incorrect treatment implemented by Ryan's doctors in response to the misdiagnosis of poisoning most likely contributed to his death.*

As in Patricia Stallings' case, inborn errors of B$_{12}$ metabolism can affect more than one child in a family. One recent report in the medical literature[23] describes two siblings, a sixteen-year-old girl and her twenty-four-year-old sister, who both suffered from methylmalonic acidemia. The younger sister became psychotic, developed severe neuropathy, and eventually was placed on a ventilator, but she recovered fully after a correct diagnosis and treatment. Her older sister suffered for two years with painful, progressive spinal cord damage before being accurately diagnosed. (The older sister's case is another example of a B$_{12}$-related problem that could easily be misdiagnosed as multiple sclerosis.) Another report by a separate group of researchers[24] describes two siblings who died as a result of undiagnosed methylmalonic aciduria, one misdiagnosed as having metabolic acidosis due to new-onset diabetes and the other misdiagnosed as having Reye's syndrome.

Clinicians should consider inborn errors of B$_{12}$ metabolism as a possibility in patients who are critically ill with unclear clinical and biochemical findings, particularly when there is a suspicious family history. Detecting such errors early can save lives and prevent disability, and, thus, prevent multiple tragedies.

Speculation: Is there an autism/B$_{12}$ connection?

Children with autism, a once-rare developmental disorder that is now becoming alarmingly common, exhibit severe speech and language problems, aloofness or abnormal social interaction, repetitive and ritualistic behavior (such as obsessively lining up toys), and in many cases self-injurious or aggressive behavior.

Some cases of autism have known causes—for instance, prenatal rubella infection, meningitis during early development, or specific genetic disorders. In general, however, autism is simply a *description* rather than an actual diagnosis, because the cause of a child's autistic symptoms is rarely identified. In fact, autism appears to have multiple causes, and preliminary clinical evidence strongly indicates that some of these causes involve inborn errors of B$_{12}$ metabolism or B$_{12}$ malabsorption in childhood.

Increasingly, doctors are finding that many autistic children improve remarkably when they receive B$_{12}$ injections. British researcher Dr. Ray Bhatt, for instance, has reported remarkable improvement in autistic children treated with vitamin B$_{12}$, saying, "The number who have benefited is a surprise."[25] Sidney Baker, M.D., a leading autism expert, notes that parents often see positive changes within "hours to days" after beginning B$_{12}$ injections, and recommends that all autistic children be screened for high MMA or other evidence of B$_{12}$ deficiency. "But even those without the MMA marker often respond dramatically to B$_{12}$," he says.[26]

James Neubrander, M.D., administered injections of methylcobalamin (methyl-B$_{12}$) to eighty-five children with autism spectrum disorders, and reports that in 50 percent of the cases, parents reported improvement in fifteen or more symptoms.[27] Arnold Brenner, M.D., who has conducted trials of injected B$_{12}$ on a number of autistic patients, says the benefits seen in his patients included decreases in hyperactivity, improvements in speech, and a reduction in anger and rage reactions. Brenner says that while two of his patients had borderline levels of B$_{12}$, most who improved had normal or even high levels, and "there are no clear biological markers as to who may benefit."[28]

It is interesting, too, that the known symptoms of pediatric B$_{12}$ deficiency include a number of symptoms resembling those of autism. Infants and children with B$_{12}$ deficiency often exhibit aloofness, a loss of speech, a loss of social skills, and movement abnormalities similar to the unusual movements seen in autism.

Autism is a complex disorder, involving genetic, infectious, autoimmune, and environmental factors, and it's highly unlikely that vitamin B$_{12}$ plays a role in every case. But Dr. Bernard Rimland, director of the Autism Research Institute and a leading international expert on the link between vitamin deficiencies and autism, says, "In my view, vitamin B$_{12}$ represents one of the most promising, and least-well investigated, modalities for treating autistic children."[29]

For our family, the issue of B$_{12}$ and autism took a personal turn in 1996 when my nephew Billy was born. At first a cuddly baby, Billy became resistant to hugs and cuddles as he grew older. He walked late, at fourteen months, and still wasn't talking at a year and a half.

Billy's parents took him for a speech evaluation that revealed a significant delay. Billy began speech therapy and started attending special classes at age three, but he was so disruptive that his preschool teachers couldn't handle him, finally placing him full-time in a class for autistic children. Billy avoided eye contact, rarely engaged in social interaction with other children or adults, did not play in a creative way, and did not initiate any speech or language but merely parroted what other people said (a behavior called echolalia, common in autism). A psychologist finally gave Billy a diagnosis—autism—and told his mother that there was no cure. His recommendation: "Make him comfortable."

Shocked by the grim outlook of the psychologist, Billy's mother took her son for additional testing by the school system and a pediatric neurologist, only to receive the same verdict: autism, with little hope for a normal or even near-normal life. Tests when Billy was four showed a slowed EEG—a sign of neurological abnormality—and a prominent rooting reflex (a reflex that is present in infants, but normally disappears around six months of age and is a sign of neurological damage when it occurs after that time).

When Billy was nearly four years old, his maternal grandmother was diagnosed with pernicious anemia. At this time, I prompted Billy's mother and father to have him tested for B$_{12}$ deficiency. We knew that his tests would be skewed, because his mother had started Billy on daily liquid B vitamins when he was just over three years old. (He had initially demonstrated small improvements in language and behavior when taking these vitamins, but his progress had leveled off.) Billy's serum B$_{12}$ levels came back high, and his Hcy level came back normal, but his MMA came back borderline high. This was fascinating, because with his high B$_{12}$ intake, his plasma MMA should have been in the very low range.

As a result of this finding, Billy's family decided to do a trial of injected B$_{12}$ (hydroxocobalamin). They did not inform family and friends, or Billy's teachers, because they wanted to receive unbiased feedback about the results—if any.

Within two weeks, the people around Billy witnessed dramatic changes. Billy started looking directly at people. His enunciation, voice tone, and verbal expressiveness improved, and he even developed a sense of humor. He started showing imagination in his play, parking his toy truck next to him at snack time and tucking in his stuffed bear in at night. He could hold a pencil, using it to draw and color, and his "chicken scratches" turned into legible letters. He stopped walking on his toes, and he no longer walked and ran with an abnormal posture. Moreover, his once-prominent abnormal rooting reflex disappeared.

After nine months of injected hydroxocobalamin (B$_{12}$), Billy entered a regular kindergarten class—a major victory for a child who was once diagnosed as incurably disabled, and whose language and behavior before the B$_{12}$ injections were equivalent developmentally to an eighteen-month-old child's. He continues to receive B$_{12}$ injections every three weeks, but no longer takes the other oral vitamin supplements, which proved unnecessary in his case. At age seven and a half, he is a year ahead of his classmates in reading and math, but one to two years behind in social skills. Labeled as autistic just a few years ago, Billy now is improving so rapidly that his parents have hope that he will lead a normal or near-normal life.

Billy's dramatic turnaround proved that he didn't suffer from incurable autism; he suffered from a B$_{12}$ deficiency, probably genetically influenced, that could be treated and at least partially (and perhaps wholly) cured with a simple monthly shot.

How many children like Billy could be helped by B$_{12}$ treatment? Currently we have no way of knowing, because to date no formal research has examined this question. But with autism now affecting as many as one in 150 children according to a recent CDC study, it is a question we urgently need to answer.

Meanwhile, any child labeled with an autism spectrum disorder should be evaluated for B$_{12}$ deficiency, using urinary MMA and plasma homocysteine tests. Because a number of autistic children with normal test results respond strongly to B$_{12}$, we also strongly recommend that every autistic child—regardless of test results—receive a trial of injected B$_{12}$ (see Chapter 12 for more information). Not every child will benefit—but for those who do, the benefits may be remarkable.

Red Flags of B$_{12}$ Deficiency
in Infants, Children, and Teenagers

If your child exhibits any of the following signs or symptoms, insist that your doctor order urinary MMA and plasma homocysteine tests:

- movement problems, including difficulty in walking or writing
- mental changes—irritability, altered mood, poor memory, "flat" emotional tone, autistic-like withdrawal
- vision problems/abnormalities
- slowed weight and height gain
- leg pains or other abnormal sensations
- fatigue
- enlarged, smooth, beefy red tongue, which may be painful or sore
- loss of previously acquired speech, language, motor, and/or social skills
- loss of appetite
- an abnormally small head circumference in infants or toddlers
- apathy, lethargy, or irritability
- involuntary movements, such as arm waving in infants or toddlers
- gray hairs/premature graying
- areas of hypopigmented skin in a Caucasian child and/or vitiligo, or areas of hyperpigmented skin in an African-American child
- rooting reflex after eight months of age (this reflex is usually absent after six months of age)

Continued on next page

Notes

1. Graham, S. M., Arvela, O. M., and Wise, G. A. Long-term neurologic consequences of nutritional vitamin B$_{12}$ deficiency in infants. *Journal of Pediatrics* 1992, 121:710–4.

2. Steen, M. T., Boddie, A. M., Fisher, A. J., Macmahon, W., Saxe, D., Sullivan, K. M., Dembure, P. P., and Elsas, L. J. Neural-tube defects are associated with low concentrations of cobalamin (vitamin B$_{12}$) in amniotic fluid. *Prenatal Diagnosis* 1998, 18(6):545–55; and, Dawson, E. B., Evans, D. R., and Van Hook, J. W. Amniotic fluid B$_{12}$ and folate levels associated with neural tube defects. *American Journal of Perinatology* 1998, 15(9):511–4; and, Thorand, B., Pietrzik, K., Prinze-Langenohl, R., Hages, M., and Holzgreve, W. Maternal and fetal serum and red blood cell folate and vitamin B$_{12}$ concentrations in pregnancies affected by neural tube defects. *Zeitschrift fur Geburtshilfe und Neonatologie* 1996, 200(5):176–80; and, Kirke, P. N., Molloy, A. M., Daly, L. E., Burke, H.,

Also insist on testing if your child:

• has undergone any surgery (including dental surgeries) involving nitrous oxide. This substance, used as an anesthetic agent and often administered during dental work or surgeries, such as insertion of ear tubes in children with chronic ear infections, can inactivate the body's stores of B$_{12}$ and cause severe neurological damage (see chapters 8 and 12)

• exhibits failure to thrive (poor appetite, poor growth and/or weight gain, general poor health)

• has a diagnosis of autism, mental retardation, developmental delay, learning disability, or neurological disorder

• has severe food allergies or sensitivities

• is diagnosed with celiac disease or gluten enteropathy

• has a thyroid or other autoimmune disorder

• has suffered a stroke or is diagnosed as having atherosclerosis

• is diagnosed with any psychiatric or behavioral disorder or problem (schizophrenia, depression, bipolar disorder, suicidal behavior, conduct disorder, anxiety disorder, attention deficit hyperactivity disorder, learning disability, etc.)

Weir, D. G., and Scott, J. M. Maternal plasma folate and vitamin B$_{12}$ are independent risk factors for neural tube defects. *Quarterly Journal of Medicine* 1993, 86(11):703–8; and, Weeks, E. W., Tamura, T., Davis, R. O., Birch, R., Vaughn, W. H., Franklin, J. C., Barganier, C., Cosper, P., Finley, S. C., and Finley, W. H. Nutrient levels in amniotic fluid from women with normal and neural tube defect pregnancies. *Biology of the Neonate* 1992, 61(4):226–31.

3. Ramakrishna, T. Vitamins and brain development. *Physiological Research* 1999, 48(3):175–87.

4. Shojania, A. M. Folic acid and vitamin B$_{12}$ deficiency in pregnancy and in the neonatal period. *Clinics in Perinatology* 1984, 11(2):433–59.

5. Davis, J. R., Goldenring, J., and Lubin, B. H. Nutritional vitamin B$_{12}$ deficiency in infants. *American Journal of Diseases of Children* 1981, 135:566–567.

6. Graham, S. M., Arvela, O. M., and Wise, G. A. Long-term neurologic consequences of nutritional vitamin B$_{12}$ deficiency in infants. *Journal of Pediatrics* 1992, 121:710–4.

7. Crane, M. G., Register, U. D., Lukens, R. H., and Gregory, R. Cobalamin (CBL) studies on two total vegetarian (vegan) families. *Vegetarian Nutrition: An International Journal* 1998, 2(3):87–92.

8. Watanabe, F., Katsura, H., Takenaka, S., Fujita, T., Abe, K., Tamura, Y., Nakatsuka, T., and Nakano, Y. Pseudovitamin B(12) is the predominant

cobamide of an algal health food, spirulina tablets. *Journal of Agricultural and Food Chemistry* 1999, 47(11):4736–41. See also: Vegetarian Society UK fact sheet, "Vitamin B$_{12}$," http://www.vegsoc.org/info/b12.html.

9. Byrne, S. "The myths of vegetarianism," *Nexus Magazine*, 2002 (online).

10. Davis, J. R., Goldenring, J., and Lubin, B. H. Nutritional vitamin B$_{12}$ deficiency in infants. *American Journal of Diseases of Children* 1981, 135:566–567.

11. Krajcovicova-Kudlackova, M., Blazicek, P., Babinska, K., Kopcova, J., Klvanova, J., Bederova, A., and Magalova, T. Traditional and alternative nutrition—levels of homocysteine and lipid parameters in adults. *Scandinavian Journal of Clinical and Laboratory Investigation* 2000, 60(8):657–64.

12. Herrmann, W., Schorr, H., Purschwitz, K., Rassoul, F., and Richter, V. Total homocysteine, vitamin B(12), and total antioxidant status in vegetarians. *Clinical Chemistry* 2001, 47(6):1094–101.

13. Bissoli, L., Di Francesco, V., Ballarin, A., Mandragona, R., Trespidi, R., Brocco, G., Caruso, B., Bosello, O., and Zamboni, M. Effect of vegetarian diet on homocysteine levels. *Annals of Nutrition and Metabolism* 2002, 46(2):73–9.

14. Crane, M. G., Register, U. D., Lukens, R. H., and Gregory, R. Cobalamin (CBL) studies on two total vegetarian (vegan) families. *Vegetarian Nutrition: An International Journal* 1998, 2(3):87–92.

15. Bjorke Monsen, A-L., Ueland, P. M., Vollset, S. E., Guttormsen, A. B., Markestad, T., Solheim, E., and Refsum, H. Determinants of cobalamin status in newborns. *Pediatrics* 2001, 108(3):624–630.

16. Gadowsky, S. L., Gale, K., Wolfe, S., Jory, J., Gibson, R., and O'Connor, D. Biochemical folate, B$_{12}$, and iron status of a group of pregnant adolescents accessed through the public health system in southern Ontario. *Journal of Adolescent Health* 1995, 16:465–474.

17. Graham, S. M., Arvela, O. M., and Wise, G. A. Long-term neurologic consequences of nutritional vitamin B$_{12}$ deficiency in infants. *Journal of Pediatrics* 1992, 121:710–4.

18. Louwman, M., van Dusseldorp, M., van de Vijver, F. J. R., Thomas, C. M. G., Schneede, J., Ueland, P. M., Refsum, H., and van Staveren, W. A. Signs of impaired cognitive function in adolescents with marginal cobalamin status. *American Journal of Clinical Nutrition* 2000, 72:762–9.

19. Licht, D. J., Berry, G. T., Brooks, D. G., and Younkin, D. P. Reversible subacute combined degeneration of the spinal cord in a fourteen-year-old due to a strict vegan diet. *Clinical Pediatrics* 2001, 40(7):413–5.

20. Fuhrman's quote appears on www.breathing.com/articles/vitamin-b12-vegan.htm.

21. Cohen M. The toppling toddler. *Discover* 2001, 22(11), online.

22. Dr. Rinaldo is quoted in "Spotlight on Childhood Diseases," on the Mayo Clinic website. (Mayroclinic.com)

23. Roze, E., et al. Neuropsychiatric disturbances in presumed late-onset cobalamin C disease. *Archives of Neurology* 2003, 60(10):1457–62.

24. Ciani, F., et al. Lethal late onset cblB methylmalonic aciduria. *Critical Care Medicine* 2000, 28:2119–21.

25. Bhatt is cited in "Vitamin disorder may be key to autism," *London Daily Telegraph*, August 17, 1995.

26. Baker, Sidney, personal communication.

27. Presentation to the Defeat Autism Now! (DAN!) Conference, Philadelphia, 2003.

28. Brenner, Arnold, "Vitamin B$_{12}$ and the autism spectrum," letter to physicians and parents, June 26, 1996.

29. Rimland, B. R. personal communication, 2002.

Vitamin B_{12} and Cancer,
Impaired Immune Function,
and Autoimmune Disease

"*Diets sufficient in methyl enhancers folate, choline, and B_{12} have proved to prevent cancer not only in animals but in humans as well.*"
—Paul Frankel, Ph.D., *The Methylation Miracle* (1999)[1]

Avoiding cancer isn't just a matter of luck and genes. While your genes influence your cancer risk, your lifestyle and your diet also play a powerful preventive role—and here again, vitamin B_{12} appears to be crucial. As we'll explain in this chapter, evidence indicates that healthy B_{12} levels can protect you against destructive processes that can contribute to cancer and to other deadly diseases as well.

The growing data on B_{12} deficiency and cancer

It's long been known that pernicious anemia, one form of B_{12} deficiency, is linked to an increased risk of gastric cancer. In this case, both the cancer and the anemia stem from an autoimmune process in which the body attacks its own cells, causing damage to parietal cells in the stomach. These cells are then unable to produce intrinsic factor (needed to metabolize B_{12}) and hydrochloric acid (needed for normal gastric function). The result: both B_{12} deficiency and damaged cells that are prone to turn cancerous.

It's less well known, however, that deficient B_{12} levels appear to be a risk factor for other forms of cancer that have nothing to do with pernicious anemia. Thus, people with B_{12} deficiency due to *any* cause—poor diet, malabsorption, metabolic defects, overexposure to nitrous oxide, use of medications that lower B$_{12}$ levels, etc.—could be unknowingly putting themselves at risk of developing cancer.

One of the strongest associations that scientists are identifying is between breast cancer and B$_{12}$ deficiency. In a recent study, researchers at Johns Hopkins measured the B$_{12}$ in blood samples taken from women who'd donated blood, comparing samples from 195 women who'd later developed breast cancer to samples from 195 cancer-free women. Among postmenopausal women, the researchers found, those whose B$_{12}$ levels fell into the lowest fifth were *two to four times* more likely to develop breast cancer than those in the upper four-fifths.[2]

This finding is exciting, because increasing vitamin B$_{12}$ intake is an easy lifestyle change to make. Even women who resist other lifestyle alterations that can lower breast cancer risk, such as increasing exercise, reducing alcohol intake, and reducing fat intake, could potentially re- duce their breast cancer risk simply by taking high-dose oral B$_{12}$ supple- ments (if they show no evidence of problems in metabolizing B$_{12}$) or receiving B$_{12}$ injections.*

In addition to breast cancer, other cancers are being tentatively linked by scientific studies to deficient levels of vitamin B$_{12}$. Among these are cervical cancer, lung cancer, and oral cancer (see box page 114).

Why do deficient B$_{12}$ levels appear to promote the development of cancer? One reason is that the body needs ample B$_{12}$ in order for folate to work, and one of folate's crucial jobs is to synthesize the nucleotide "building blocks" of DNA. When folate is trapped in an unusable form due to a lack of B$_{12}$, it can't do this job correctly.

This leads to an imbalance in the supply of DNA building blocks, forcing the body to make changes in DNA structure that can make the DNA more vulnerable to breakage. Broken DNA strands can lead to mu-

---

* At first glance, the finding of a link between B$_{12}$ deficiency and breast cancer seems to fly in the face of other studies reporting that vegetarians are less likely than other women to develop breast cancer. (As we've noted, B$_{12}$ occurs naturally only in animal products.) This finding initially led researchers to suggest a link between a high-meat diet and breast cancer. However, newer research clarifies the issue, showing no increased risk of breast cancer in women who eat diets high in meat (see New England Journal of Medicine HealthNews, July 2002). It is the protective effect of vegetables, fruits, legumes, and fiber that reduces breast cancer risk in vegetarian women, and not a lower intake of animal products.

tations that, in turn, can lead to cancer. Research shows that chromosome breakage is strongly correlated with deficiencies of either folate or B$_{12}$ (or with high levels of homocysteine, linked to B vitamin deficiencies), and that large dietary supplements of B$_{12}$ can minimize this breakage.[8]

Could B$_{12}$ Deficiency Increase Your Risk of Cancer?

Are you at greater risk of developing cancer if your B$_{12}$ levels are too low? Research findings indicate that the answer is a definite "yes." Among the reports are the following conclusions:

• Researchers looking at B$_{12}$ levels in women with and without cervical cancer found that both folic acid and B$_{12}$ appeared to exert protective effects.[3]

• A study of human papillomavirus (HPV) infection—an infection strongly linked to the development of cervical cancer—found that women with lower levels of B$_{12}$ circulating in their blood tended to have more persistent HPV infection.[4]

• A recent study showed that the risk of invasive cervical cancer is greatly elevated for women with high levels of homocysteine, an amino acid that damages the body when it accumulates in excess (see Chapter 5). High homocysteine levels are in turn linked to low levels of folate, vitamin B$_{12}$, and/or vitamin B$_6$.[5]

• Studying cancerous lung tissue and adjacent non-cancerous cells taken from patients with lung cancer, researchers found that folate and B$_{12}$ levels were significantly lower in cells that had turned cancerous than in adjacent, non-cancerous cells.[6]

• Researchers in Alabama studied women who were at high risk for oral cancer because they chewed tobacco or betel. Women who ate fewer servings of animal products were more likely to have pre-malignant lesions than those who ate more animal-based foods, and those eating low amounts of both animal products and vegetables were at highest risk[7] — not a surprising finding, since the B$_{12}$ from animal products and the folate from vegetables work hand-in-hand.

In addition, B$_{12}$ deficiency can cause defects in a biological process called methylation, and these defects in turn can cause the wrong genes on chromosomes to "turn on" or prevent the right genes from being activated. Abnormal methylation patterns are characteristic of cells that are in the process of turning cancerous, and scientist Sang-Woon Choi notes that "genomic DNA hypomethylation is a common phenomenon in cancers in the colon, lung, stomach, uterus, and cervix." Abnormal hypermethylation, too, is implicated in some cancers.

How important are proper methylation, and a diet high in the nutrients that your body needs for this process, in preventing cancer? One study showed that a diet high in folate, required for proper methylation, is associated with a nearly 40 percent drop in colon cancer risk. (You'll remember that folate can do its job only in the presence of B$_{12}$—so if you're B$_{12}$-deficient, much of the folate in your body is useless.) Another found that high doses of folic acid and vitamin B$_{12}$ markedly reduce the numbers of precancerous cells in the sputum of cigarette smokers. Still another study, this one in Japan, found that smokers taking supplements of B$_{12}$ and folate showed a dramatic reversal of cell changes linked to the development of cancer.[9] There's also some evidence linking poor methylation or a diet low in the nutrients that promote methylation to liver cancer, childhood brain tumors, lymphoma, and pancreatic cancer.[10]

Poor methylation also results in high levels of the amino acid homocysteine, which can put you at risk not only for heart disease (see Chapter 5) but possibly also for cancer—and, in particular, for "female" cancers. Cancer researcher B. T. Zhu notes that the high homocysteine levels resulting from low B$_{12}$, folate, and/or B$_6$ levels can cause the body to break down estrogens abnormally, reducing levels of one tumor-inhibiting estrogen metabolite while leading to an accumulation of a different one that is "strongly procarcinogenic."

"This hypothesis," he says, "...predicts that adequate dietary intake of folate, vitamin B$_6$ and vitamin B$_{12}$ may reduce hyperhomocysteinemia-associated risk for hormonal cancer."[11]

Moreover, B$_{12}$ deficiency impairs the functioning of the immune system, and an immune system that isn't functioning right can't defend you as well against cancerous cells. In fact, the immune system problems that result from B$_{12}$ deficiency are linked not just to cancer but also to a range of problems we'll discuss later in this chapter.

What Is Methylation?

Methylation is the process by which methyl groups (molecules consisting of one carbon atom and three hydrogen atoms) attach to different substances in the body, changing their function. One important job of methylation is to prevent potentially harmful genes from being expressed.

Paul Frankel, Ph.D., an expert on methylation, explains this in simple terms: "Imagine your genetic makeup as a blueprint for a house, and the methyl groups as coffee cups sitting on the blueprint. Since you can build only the part of the blueprint you see, when you put a cup in a different place, it covers up a different part of the house, and therefore that part is not made—or 'expressed' in genetic terms."

As we age, our bodies become less able to correctly methylate DNA. The result: more and more DNA errors that can eventually lead to the expression of cancer-promoting genes. Deficiencies of vitamin B$_{12}$, folic acid, vitamin B$_6$, and choline dramatically increase the risk of improper methylation, as can a high alcohol intake.

It's critical to optimize your intake of methylation-promoting nutrients *before* a cancer can develop. Improving your methylation status after a cancer develops will improve the health of all of your cells, but unfortunately that includes cancerous cells as well as normal ones.

When B$_{12}$ deficiency causes false cancer scares

In addition to increasing your risk of cancer, B$_{12}$ deficiency can increase the odds that you'll receive an *incorrect* diagnosis of precancerous lesions, particularly if you're a woman. That's because B$_{12}$ deficiency causes the cells lining the cervix to become deformed. These cell changes can cause Pap smears to appear abnormal, often leading to additional tests or even to unnecessary surgeries.

Thus, the presence of what appear to be pre-malignant cells in a Pap smear should always lead doctors to include comprehensive B$_{12}$ testing, including urinary MMA and homocysteine tests, as part of the diagnostic process.

For one fifty-seven-year-old woman we know, the diagnosis of B$_{12}$ deficiency came at least eight years too late.

Luckily, the diagnosis came in time to spare her from dementia, paralysis, pain and suffering, and early death. Although her doctors initially labeled her arm tremor and numbness as essential tremor or possibly a symptom of multiple sclerosis, her son (a physician) ordered the tests I recommended for B$_{12}$ deficiency and discovered her real diagnosis: autoimmune pernicious anemia. As a result, she won't experience the inexorable mental and physical decline that so many people with undiagnosed B$_{12}$ deficiency suffer. But she wasn't spared from years of unnecessary worry, expense, and debility that preceded her diagnosis.

Clearly, her tremor should have led to testing for B$_{12}$ deficiency, because medical texts and articles (see Chapter 3) describe the neurological consequences of this deficiency—consequences that can include tremor and numbness. In addition, this woman suffered from Hashimoto's thyroiditis, an autoimmune disorder that is strongly associated with autoimmune pernicious anemia, and her mother had been diagnosed with pernicious anemia. The most basic and inexpensive test for low B$_{12}$, a serum B$_{12}$ level (ordered later by her son), clearly showed her deficiency. The more accurate MMA test confirmed this diagnosis, and further testing revealed her autoimmune pernicious anemia.

But the problem could have been detected still earlier by other physicians, including the woman's gynecologist. She'd had abnormal Pap smears for eight years, which is not rare for B$_{12}$-deficient women because—as we've noted above—the cells that line the cervix don't form normally in the absence of adequate supplies of this vitamin. But her OB/GYN never tested her for B$_{12}$ deficiency. Instead, every six months, he ordered a repeat Pap smear (which also came back abnormal). Also, because of this woman's abnormal Pap smears, the doctor ordered a dilatation and curettage (D&C) and a loop electrosurgical excision procedure (LEEP), both unpleasant procedures. These treatments didn't eradicate her atypical cervical cells, and in addition, she suffered the mental anguish of repeated cancer scares and the strain of waiting for biopsy results.

This woman was diagnosed with pernicious anemia in July of 2000, began receiving injections of B$_{12}$, and went back to her OB/GYN for a repeat Pap smear in October. This time, for the first time in eight years, the result was perfectly normal. This doesn't surprise us at all, because her untreated pernicious anemia made the cells irregular in the first *place—and treating that disease caused the cells to become healthy again.*

Suggesting that the test results "could be an error," her OB/GYN recommended that she continue to have biannual Pap smears. Instead, she waited a year before undergoing her next Pap smear, which once again came back perfectly normal. It is now four years since she began receiving B$_{12}$ shots, and her Pap smears continue to show no abnormalities.

It's possible that the abnormal cervical cells seen in women with B$_{12}$ deficiency could eventually become cancerous, if the deficiency is not treated in time. (The strong association between B$_{12}$ deficiency and cervical cancer certainly suggests this.) Thus, doctors who consider possible B$_{12}$ deficiency in all patients with abnormal Pap smears will not only save B$_{12}$-deficient women time, money, and stress—they may also save some of these women's lives.

B$_{12}$'s effects on immune function

One consequence of an immune system damaged by low B$_{12}$ is cancer. But the immune system that's too low in B$_{12}$ can go awry in many ways, and the results can take many forms—most of them serious, and many potentially fatal.

For example, B$_{12}$ deficiency appears to make the body react abnormally to vaccines, a problem that can be life threatening. Evidence of this comes from a recent study of elderly hospital patients given a vaccine to protect against pneumonia. (This is the same shot that seniors routinely receive.) Half of the participants had very low B$_{12}$ levels, while the other half—matched for age and diagnosis—had higher levels.

Before receiving the shots, both groups of patients had similar levels of antibodies to pneumonia. Afterward, however, the group with high B$_{12}$ levels had much higher antibody levels than those with low B$_{12}$ levels. This indicates, the researchers say, that while vaccination leads to the formation of "memory cells" primed to combat disease, the development of these cells into an effective disease-fighting force depends in part on the level of vitamin B$_{12}$.

"These findings may be clinically significant," according to the researchers, "since the efficacy of the pneumococcal vaccine is only about 46 to 70 percent in the elderly, and a significant proportion of elderly patients have subclinical vitamin B$_{12}$ deficiency."[12] Translation: If you're a senior citizen who's careful to get your pneumonia vaccination, you may be wasting your money if you're low in B$_{12}$, because the shot might not protect you at all.

Moreover, since any vaccination can adversely affect individuals with impaired immune systems, we speculate that B$_{12}$ deficiency may play a key role in some of the thousands of severe reactions to immunizations that occur each year. Given the findings in the pneumonia vaccine study, this is an area that requires further serious study.

HIV, AIDS, and B$_{12}$

AIDS (acquired immunodeficiency syndrome), a disease that cripples the immune system and leaves its victims defenseless against many infections and cancers, is caused by the human immunodeficiency virus, or HIV. Growing evidence shows that B$_{12}$ deficiency is extremely common in individuals with AIDS, and this deficiency may play a role in the progress of the disease.

One remarkable finding is that B$_{12}$ deficiency is linked to a more rapid onset of AIDS symptoms in people who've been infected with HIV. Researchers at Johns Hopkins discovered that whether or not participants were undergoing prescription drug treatment, "development of deficiency of vitamin A or vitamin B$_{12}$ was associated with a decline in CD4 cell count, while normalization of vitamin A, vitamin B$_{12}$ and zinc was associated with higher CD4 cell counts." The researchers conclude, "These data suggest that micronutrient deficiencies are associated with HIV-1 disease progression and raise the possibility that normalization might increase symptom-free survival."[13] A similar study, by a different research group, found that HIV-infected men with low serum B$_{12}$ levels "had significantly shorter AIDS-free time" than those with adequate B$_{12}$ levels.[14]

In related research, investigators discovered that under experimental conditions, several forms of vitamin B$_{12}$ (including methylcobalamin and hydroxocobalamin) inhibit HIV infection of blood cells. The researchers suggest that "these or related agents may be useful as anti-viral treatments" that target HIV.[15]

Low B$_{12}$ levels are very common in HIV-infected individuals, with up to a third showing signs of deficiency, and about half showing evidence of low B$_{12}$,[16] often in spite of normal serum B$_{12}$ levels. One reason for this deficiency is that patients with AIDS-related diarrhea absorb vitamin B$_{12}$ very poorly.[17] Another is that AIDS patients exhibit reductions in stomach acid, intrinsic factor, and holotranscobalamin II (substances needed to break down B$_{12}$, transport it to the intestine, and carry it to cells throughout the body).[18]

It is possible that B$_{12}$ plays a significant role in the neurological symptoms associated with AIDS. Almost a third of people with AIDS suffer from neuropathy, a painful tingling or numbness of the feet, legs, arms, or hands. This neuropathy is very similar to that seen in patients with a primary diagnosis of B$_{12}$ deficiency (see Chapter 3). HIV-related neuropathy can stem from a number of causes, including the use of medications such as Hivid, Videx, Zerit, Epivir, dapsone, Myambutol, isoniazid, Flagyl, Taxol, Thalomid, or Oncovin (some of which, by the way, also reduce B$_{12}$ levels). However, given the high incidence of B$_{12}$ deficiency in people with AIDS, depleted B$_{12}$ stores may very well contribute to a significant number of cases of HIV-related neuropathy.

Even in AIDS patients whose B$_{12}$ levels appear normal, the body's B$_{12}$ pathways can break down in ways that lead to neurological problems. One group of scientists recently studied patients with AIDS and myelopathy (nervous system damage), patients with AIDS but without myelopathy, and non-HIV-infected controls. The AIDS patients with myelopathy, but not those free of this symptom, showed defects in a crucial B$_{12}$ pathway. This is additional strong evidence that "hidden" B$_{12}$ problems are common in AIDS, and these problems could cause or worsen neurological symptoms in many AIDS patients.

Another terrifying symptom of AIDS is dementia, which often occurs in late stages of the disease. Here again, it's possible that B$_{12}$ deficiency is part of the picture. As we explained in Chapter 2, B$_{12}$ deficiency is strongly linked to dementia in the elderly—so it makes sense that the rampant B$_{12}$ deficiency in AIDS patients may contribute to dementia in this group as well.

Future research will give us a better understanding of the possible link between AIDS symptoms and B$_{12}$ deficiency. In the meantime, because the B$_{12}$ pathways can break down at so many stages in AIDS, we strongly recommend that anyone with HIV or AIDS receive regular injections of vitamin B$_{12}$ or take a high daily dose of oral methylcobalamin.

George, a thirty-eight-year-old diagnosed with AIDS, visited our ER three times in two months complaining of painful foot neuropathy. I reviewed his blood work and noted that no doctor had ordered a serum B$_{12}$ level, much less an MMA. Instead, his physicians had treated his painful neuropathy with Neurontin (which was ineffective), telling him there was nothing more they could do.

I told George to get his MMA and B$_{12}$ levels checked, but his doctors did not follow through on this advice. Recently, I came across his chart, and I found that he'd returned to the ER two years after I'd last seen him. At the most recent visit, he was anemic, his blood smear showed signs of B$_{12}$ deficiency, and his gastroenterologist reported that an endoscopy of his stomach showed atrophic gastritis (inflammation and wasting of the stomach lining that drastically decreases stomach acid, impairing the body's ability to break B$_{12}$ apart from protein so it can be absorbed).

George is still taking Neurontin, even though it barely takes the edge off his pain. His doctors also put him on Prevacid, which will reduce his stomach acid still further and worsen his already-serious B$_{12}$ depletion. Given his obvious B$_{12}$ deficiency, it is likely that this treatment will put him at risk for increasing motor problems, pain, and eventually dementia.

B$_{12}$ deficiency and autoimmune disorders

It seems strange that B$_{12}$ deficiency is involved in both under-activation and over-activation of the immune system. But it's true, because in addition to being linked to poor disease resistance, B$_{12}$ deficiency is linked to autoimmune disorders in which the body attacks its own cells.

Pernicious anemia is a condition in which the stomach lining that contains the parietal cells is destroyed through an autoimmune mechanism. The parietal cells secrete intrinsic factor, which is necessary for B$_{12}$ absorption. Without intrinsic factor, B$_{12}$ deficiency ensues. It is thought that this failure of intrinsic factor secretion is a result of gastric mucosal atrophy (wasting of the stomach lining). The gastric atrophy is caused from immune destruction of the acid and pepsin secreting portions of the stomach lining. Pernicious anemia patients have poor gastric acid production and often complain of a bloated and prolonged full feeling after eating. Progressive destruction of the parietal cells causes decreased secretion of hydrochloric acid and enzymes required to release

Aids in Africa: a B$_{12}$ Link?

AIDS is a worldwide problem, but it strikes African nations the hardest. There are many reasons for this, including poverty and lack of health education. However, it's our guess that B$_{12}$ deficiency could possibly play at least some role in the AIDS crisis in African countries.

Many Africans eat a mostly vegetarian diet lacking in B$_{12}$.[19] In addition, most African women breast-feed their children, which is a good idea when maternal diets are adequate, but can lead to drastically low B$_{12}$ levels in children when mothers have B$_{12}$ deficiency. And, malnutrition is rampant in many areas of Africa, with one study showing that children in a rural South African community had dietary intakes below 50 percent of the RDA for vitamin B$_{12}$ and a host of other nutrients.[20]

Given that B$_{12}$ deficiency impairs the immune system's ability to fight off infection, and may speed the development of AIDS in HIV-infected people, it is only logical to assume that the poor B$_{12}$ status of millions of Africans could play a role in this terrible epidemic. It would be wise for the public health officials combating this crisis to include, as part of their prevention strategy, efforts to improve the B$_{12}$ status of people throughout Africa.

food-bound vitamin B$_{12}$. Over time, this leads to wasting and inflammation of the stomach lining and achlorhydria (no stomach acid). Typically, antibodies to parietal cells and/or intrinsic factor are seen in pernicious anemia patients. The term pernicious anemia is often used as a synonym for B$_{12}$ deficiency, but it should be reserved for the autoimmune condition.

A person with one autoimmune disorder is at a higher risk for other autoimmune disorders. For instance, autoimmune thyroid disorders (Hashimoto's thyroiditis, Graves' disease) and type 1 diabetes are common in B$_{12}$-deficient individuals. Other autoimmune disorders associated with pernicious anemia include Addison's disease, vitiligo, premature ovarian failure, rheumatoid arthritis, lupus, hypoparathyroidism, hypogammaglobulinemia, agammaglobulinemia, ulcerative colitis, and idiopathic adrenocortical insufficiency. Therefore, patients with pernicious anemia should be screened for other autoimmune disorders, especially disorders of the thyroid.

Is low B$_{12}$ putting you at risk for cancer or other immune-related problems?

Research suggests that B$_{12}$ deficiency may increase any individual's risk for immune system dysfunction or cancer, but you may be particularly vulnerable if:

- You have an autoimmune disorder
- You have a family history of autoimmune disorders or impaired immune system function
- You have a family history of cancer, and in particular gastrointestinal or "female" cancers
- You have a history of abnormal Pap smears
- You carry the HIV virus or have AIDS

Notes

1. Frankel, P. *The Methylation Miracle*, New York: St. Martin's Press, 1999.
2. Wu, K., Helzlsouer, K. J., Comstock, G. W., Hoffman, S. C., Nadeau, M. R., and Selhub, J. A prospective study on folate, B$_{12}$, and pyridoxal 5'-phosphate (B6) and breast cancer. *Cancer Epidemiology, Biomarkers and Prevention* 1999, 8(3):209–17.
3. Alberg, A. J., Selhub, J., Shah, K. V., Viscidi, R. P., Comstock, G. W., and Helzlsouer, K. J. The risk of cervical cancer in relation to serum concentrations of folate, vitamin B$_{12}$, and homocysteine. *Cancer Epidemiology, Biomarkers, and Prevention* 2000, 9(7):761–4.
4. Sedjo, R. L., Inserra, P., Abrahamsen, M., Harris, R. B., Roe, D. J., Baldwin, S., and Giuliano, A. R. Human papillomavirus persistence and nutrients involved in the methylation pathway among a cohort of young women. *Cancer Epidemiology, Biomarkers and Prevention* 2002, 11(4):353–9.
5. Weinstein, S. J., Ziegler, R. G., Selhub, J., Fears, T. R., Strickler, H. D., Brinton, L. A., Hamman, R. F., Levine, R. S., Mallin, K., and Stolley, P. D. Elevated serum homocysteine levels and increased risk of invasive cervical cancer in US women. *Cancer Causes and Control* 2001, 12(4):317–24.
6. Piyathilake, C. J., Johanning, G. L., Macaluso, M., Whiteside, M., Oelschlager, D. K., Heimburger, D. C., and Grizzle, W. E. Localized folate and vitamin B-12 deficiency in squamous cell lung cancer is associated with global DNA hypomethylation. *Nutrition and Cancer* 2000, 37(1):99–107.
7. Carley, K. W., Puttaiah, R., Alvarez, J. O., Heimburger, D. C., and Anantha, N. Diet and oral premalignancy in female south Indian tobacco and betel chewers: A case-control study. *Nutr Cancer* 1994, 22(1):73–84.
8. Choi, Sang-Woon. Vitamin B$_{12}$ deficiency: A new risk factor for breast cancer? *Nutrition Reviews* 1999, 57(8):250–53.
9. All three studies cited in Frankel, P., *The Methylation Miracle*, New York: St. Martin's Press, 1999.
10. Frankel, P. *The Methylation Miracle*. New York: St. Martin's Press, 1999.
11. Zhu, B. T. Medical hypothesis: Hyperhomocysteinemia is a risk factor for estrogen-induced hormonal cancer. *International Journal of Oncology* 2003, 22(3):499–508.
12. Fata, F., Herzlich, B., Schiffman, G., and Ast, A. Impaired antibody responses to pneumococcal polysaccharide in elderly patients with low serum vitamin B$_{12}$ levels. *Annals of Internal Medicine* 1996, 124:299–304.
13. Baum, M. K., Shor-Posner, G., Lu, Y., Rosner, B., Sauberlich, H. E., Fletcher, M. A., Szapocznik, J., Eisdorfer, C., Buring, J. E., and Hennekens, C. H. *AIDS* 1995, 9(9):1051–6.
14. Tang, A. M., Graham, N. M., Chandra, R. K., and Saah, A. J. Low serum vitamin B$_{12}$ concentrations are associated with faster human immunodeficiency virus type 1 (HIV-1) disease progression. *Journal of Nutrition*

1997, 127(2):345–51.

15. Weinberg, J. B., Shugars, D. C., Sherman, P. A., Sauls, D. L., and Fyfe, J. A. Cobalamin inhibition of HIV-1 integrase and integration of HIV-1 DNA into cellular DNA. *Biochemical and Biophysical Research Communications* 1998, 246(2):393–7.

16. Herbert, V., Fong, W., Gulle, V., and Stopler, T. Low holotranscobalamin II is the earliest serum marker for subnormal vitamin B$_{12}$ (cobalamin) absorption in patients with AIDS. *American Journal of Hematology* 1990, 34(2):132–9.

17. Bjarnason, I., Sharpstone, D. R., Francis, N., Marker, A., Taylor, C., Barrett. M., Macpherson, A., Baldwin, C., Menzies, I. S., Crane, R. C., Smith, T., Pozniak, A., and Gazzard, B. G. Intestinal inflammation, ileal structure and function in HIV. *AIDS* 1996, 10(12):1385–91.

18. Herzlich, B. C., Schiano, T. D., Moussa, Z., Zimbalist, E., Panagopoulos, G., Ast, A., and Nawabi, I. Decreased intrinsic factor secretion in AIDS: Relation to parietal cell acid secretory capacity and vitamin B$_{12}$ malabsorption. *American Journal of Gastroenterology* 1992, 87(12):1781–8.

19. Neumann, C. G. Livestock development and impact on diet quality and the growth and development of children. Consultative Group on International Agricultural Research, http://www.cgiar.org.

20. Faber, M., Jogessar, V. B., and Benade, A. J. Nutritional status and dietary intakes of children aged 2–5 years and their caregivers in a rural South African community. *International Journal of Food Science and Nutrition* 2001, 52(5):401–11.

Under the Knife: Why Low B_{12} Levels Make Surgery Dangerous

Imagine how it feels to hear that your tiny, beautiful four-month-old baby needs an operation. Luckily, the doctor tells you the problem is correctable: The bones of her skull fused too early, and the surgeon needs to remove some tissue so her brain has room to grow.

On the day of the surgery, you kiss your daughter looking impossibly tiny and helpless as she's wheeled off to the operating room. You will the clock to move faster as the minutes tick by, telling yourself that nothing will go wrong, that she's going to be fine. Eventually, you breathe a sigh of relief when the surgeon comes through the doors and tells you that all went well.

But later on, you find out that it didn't. Your baby, happy and healthy before her surgery, stops smiling and loses her sparkle and playfulness. She also stops eating, grows "floppy" and unresponsive, and becomes so dehydrated that she needs emergency treatment. In the hospital, magnetic resonance imaging scans reveal brain atrophy. Tests show that your baby's B_{12} stores dropped to dangerous levels after the anesthetic agent used in her surgery severely worsened her undetected B_{12} deficiency. Now she's desperately ill, and she may never fully recover.

No surgery, minor or major, is risk-free. Even if you're in the hands of the best doctors, and the best operating room staffs, unpredictable crises can occur, and there's a chance you may become crippled or even die. It's a risk you're likely willing to take, if an operation can improve or even save your life.

Surgery can be vastly more risky, however, if you're one of the millions of Americans who suffer from undiagnosed B$_{12}$ deficiency. In fact, if you're B$_{12}$-deficient, even the simplest of surgical or dental procedures can turn dangerous or even deadly—and your doctor or dentist isn't likely to recognize that you're at risk until it's too late.

The danger to B$_{12}$-deficient surgery patients involves a very common anesthetic agent, nitrous oxide (N$_2$O), used millions of times a year to reduce pain and sedate patients during surgical and dental procedures. You probably know this agent better as "laughing gas," because of its well-known ability to make you feel giggly—an effect that makes it a popular drug of abuse. For people with undiagnosed B$_{12}$ deficiency, however, there's nothing funny about N$_2$O's effects. That's because nitrous oxide has an unusual side effect: It inactivates vitamin B$_{12}$ in the body.

If you're not B$_{12}$-deficient, this typically isn't dangerous, because your body can renew its stores of B$_{12}$ within a few days. But if your B$_{12}$ levels are too low, or you have an undetected B$_{12}$ malabsorption problem, exposure to nitrous oxide during surgery can have devastating consequences—even if you're young or middle-aged, and even if you're perfectly healthy before undergoing your surgery.

The story that begins this chapter, based on a real-life case,[1] is a good example. This four-month-old baby appeared healthy and normal before her surgery, despite her undetected B$_{12}$ deficiency. Now, as a result of the neurological damage she suffered when exposure to N$_2$O inactivated her already-low B$_{12}$ stores, she may be mentally disabled for life. Other B$_{12}$-deficient patients lose their ability to walk, suffer excruciating pain, become paralyzed or incontinent, or even develop full-blown dementia after exposure to N$_2$O.

Nitrous oxide's ability to wreak havoc on the mind and body of a B$_{12}$-deficient patient isn't a new discovery. Doctors first reported the phenomenon a quarter-century ago, and dozens of case studies are described in the medical literature. Moreover, it's not just a handful of patients who are at risk. Neurosurgeons Kathryn Holloway and Anthony Alberico say, "N$_2$O is very dangerous in the B$_{12}$-deficient patient. Because B$_{12}$ deficiency is not uncommon and N$_2$O use is ubiquitous, the potential exists in every [surgical] practice for this complication to occur." Thus, they stress, "The surgeon should... look for evidence of B$_{12}$ deficiency in every patient."[2]

Unfortunately, most surgeons don't, and the consequences of this failure can be horrific.

A sixty-nine-year-old retired butcher undergoes what should be a routine surgery for a benign prostate problem. Within two weeks, he finds it increasingly hard to walk, and his legs become numb.

About this time, he develops gallbladder problems, and his doctors admit him for a second surgery. Despite the patient's bad reaction to his first surgery—a likely indication of deficient B$_{12}$ stores—his doctors again use N$_2$O. After the surgery, he becomes confused, and the numbness in his legs grows worse. Within four months, he's paralyzed from the waist down and can barely use his arms. He becomes incontinent, and he suffers from memory loss, disorientation, and other symptoms resembling senile dementia.

It takes three months for the man's doctors to diagnose the cause of his paralysis and mental deterioration. He starts B$_{12}$ therapy, but it's too late to reverse his symptoms fully, and even after an entire year of treatment and physical therapy, he can walk unaided only for short distances.[3]

This patient suffered terribly when doctors exposed him to N$_2$O without discovering his preexisting B$_{12}$ deficiency. Yet his doctors did everything "by the book"—because "the book" doesn't say anything about testing patients for B$_{12}$ deficiency before they undergo surgery.

This probably surprises you if you've had surgery, because your doctor undoubtedly ordered an alphabet soup of impressive-looking tests before your operation—CBC, LYTES, BUN, CREAT, PT/PTT, etc. Look at the list, however, and you'll probably find that serum B$_{12}$, the most basic test for B$_{12}$ deficiency, isn't on it. Neither, predictably, will be the urinary MMA, the more accurate identifier of hidden B$_{12}$ deficiency.

Some doctors do give patients single injections of B$_{12}$ before procedures involving N$_2$O, to reduce the risk of a dangerous reaction in anyone who might have low B$_{12}$ stores. However, this "one-shot" approach probably won't prevent complications in severely deficient patients who are exposed to N$_2$O for several hours. It also fails to identify preoperative B$_{12}$ deficiencies that will continue to cause insidious damage and may have contributed to the disorders that led to the need for surgery in the first place. Also, giving an undiagnosed patient a single shot of B$_{12}$ can cloud the results of future lab tests, leaving doctors unable to identify a deficiency, if one exists.

Why don't doctors and dentists test for B$_{12}$ deficiency before a surgery? One reason is cost, because screening could add one hundred dollars or so to your insurance company's tab. Another reason is that many doctors assume, wrongly, that standard pre-surgical blood work will turn up any B$_{12}$ problems. And still another reason is ignorance: Many doctors and dentists simply aren't aware of the risks of administering N$_2$O to B$_{12}$-deficient patients. In addition, even doctors who know about N$_2$O's potential negative effects on patients with B$_{12}$ deficiency tend to think that bad reactions, as well as B$_{12}$ deficiency itself, are extremely rare. But on this point, the doctors are almost certainly wrong.

Tip of the iceberg?

In one small way, patients with severe reactions to N$_2$O are lucky: Because their symptoms are so drastic, many eventually do receive a diagnosis of B$_{12}$ deficiency—although in some cases it takes months, and the diagnosis often comes too late to fully restore their health.

But what about patients who suffer side effects that are dismissed as "typical" or "not unexpected" after a surgical procedure? Millions of patients deteriorate after undergoing cardiac bypass surgery, cancer surgery, or other operations. Among the most common problems we see in postoperative patients are the following:

- depression
- strokes
- memory loss
- fatigue
- falls
- neuropathies or unexplained pains
- confusion
- weakness
- transient ischemic attacks (TIAs)
- balance problems
- dizziness

The medical profession tends to assume that these are sad but common and unavoidable risks of surgery, especially in seniors or patients undergoing back surgery or neurological procedures. But what's interesting is that all of these symptoms can also be symptoms of B$_{12}$ deficiency. Of course, patients suffer postoperative problems for many reasons, and B$_{12}$ deficiency is just one of them. But consider that as many as a third of all adults are at least marginally B$_{12}$ deficient, and approximately 15 percent of seniors (and up to 40 percent of seniors with significant health problems, who are the most common candidates for surgery) are seriously deficient. This adds up to a huge number of at-risk patients.

Now, consider that U.S. hospitals perform more than 41 million inpatient surgical operations each year, many involving N$_2$O—yet these hospitals screen only a handful of patients for B$_{12}$ deficiency. Dentists also perform millions of in-office surgical procedures each year, many of them involving N$_2$O, and yet few check to determine if patients have a history or signs and symptoms of B$_{12}$ deficiency.

All of this—millions of high-risk patients, millions of surgeries using N$_2$O, and a virtual lack of B$_{12}$ screening—creates a huge potential for serious, life-threatening side effects. Anesthesiologist Jonny Hobbhahn notes that when you add to this equation the fact that symptoms often take weeks to develop, it's reasonable to assume that there is "a greater incidence of neurological deficits than reflected by the published cases."[4] Doctors Holloway and Alberico agree, saying, "It is tempting to speculate on how many unexpected new postoperative neurological deficits in surgical patients may have actually been due to B$_{12}$ deficiency and nitrous oxide administration."[5]

But all we can do is speculate, because the issue has never been the subject of an in-depth epidemiological investigation. Logic tells us, however, that for every patient diagnosed with obvious symptoms of B$_{12}$ depletion due to N$_2$O, many more are likely to suffer symptoms that are written off as coincidental. For a patient with borderline B$_{12}$ deficiency undergoing a short surgery, these complications could be as mild as numb or tingling legs. But a severely B$_{12}$-deficient patient who undergoes hours of surgery—say, for a heart bypass—may never wake up after the operation, or he or she may become paralyzed or appear to have suffered a stroke. Given that doctors generally don't evaluate patients' B$_{12}$ status before surgery, the likelihood of an accurate diagnosis after surgery is slim—especially when catastrophic outcomes can easily be blamed on old age or frailty.

One conclusion that isn't mere speculation is that most of the N$_2$O-caused tragedies that are reported could have been prevented. The majority of life-threatening cases described in the medical literature involved patients with known risk factors for B$_{12}$ deficiency. These patients' suffering could have been avoided if alert doctors had spotted the warning signs—slightly abnormal blood tests, preexisting neurological or gastrointestinal problems, past histories of bad reactions to surgeries involving N$_2$O, patients over the age of sixty—and ordered a couple of simple tests.

A healthy, active fifty-eight-year old woman underwent surgery for a benign abdominal mass. A month later, her feet started tingling and she began dragging her right leg when she walked. When her surgery site became infected, she underwent a second procedure, again under nitrous oxide—in spite of her bad reaction to her first surgery, which should have raised a red flag.

"In two weeks," says the physician who reported the case, "she became so unsteady on her feet that she fell backward if she closed her eyes." Within a short time, she could no longer stand without help, button her shirt, or write legibly.[6]

How can you protect yourself from N$_2$O-caused pain, paralysis, or dementia? The answer is simple. If you already know that you have a history of B$_{12}$ deficiency, refuse to allow an anesthesiologist or dentist to use N$_2$O, because there are safer and equally effective substitutes. Otherwise, calculate your risk for B$_{12}$ deficiency (see Chapter 10). If you're at elevated risk, insist on being tested for B$_{12}$ deficiency if you're scheduled for an elective surgery involving N$_2$O. Even if you aren't at higher-than-average risk, it's a good idea to be tested, especially if you're middle-aged or older.

Make sure your doctor orders not just a serum B$_{12}$ test, but also the urinary MMA test described in chapters 10 and 11. Taken together, these two tests will reliably rule out B$_{12}$ deficiency. Extra caution is called for in surgeries involving patients diagnosed with multiple sclerosis, developmental disabilities, or neurological disorders.

If you're at elevated risk, be sure to insist on testing even if a doctor or dentist tells you that your surgery will be too brief to cause problems. It's true that the longer your exposure to N$_2$O, the greater your risk, but neurologist Marie Rose-Marié warns, "In patients with borderline cobalamin (B$_{12}$) stores, even short exposures to nitrous oxide may be sufficient to precipitate a [B$_{12}$] deficiency syndrome."[7] Also, be aware that repeated surgeries, even short ones, can increase your risk of developing N$_2$O-caused neurological problems.

Don't be surprised, however, if your doctor is reluctant to order pre-surgical tests for B$_{12}$ deficiency, or even to evaluate you for it if you experience symptoms after a surgery using N$_2$O. An acquaintance of ours recently became quadriplegic after a seven-hour surgery for a herniated disc. When the man's son requested tests to rule out B$_{12}$ deficiency as a possible cause of the paralysis, the neurosurgeon refused—even when the man's wife, a registered nurse, provided the doctor with articles from medical journals describing cases of paralysis in B$_{12}$-deficient patients exposed to N$_2$O. Such egotism and opposition are particularly disturbing because, unlike many postsurgical complications, symptoms of N$_2$O-caused B$_{12}$ deficiency can be reversed—but only if they're caught quickly.

A forty-seven-year-old former ballet dancer underwent eight hours of cosmetic surgery. Her recovery went well for six weeks, but then she developed balance problems, odd sensations in her arms and legs, numbness, and weakness. She began falling, and she walked with an unsteady gait. Doctors identified her N$_2$O-caused B$_{12}$ deficiency and started her immediately on B$_{12}$ injections. Within sixteen weeks, she was back to normal, except for mild fatigue.[8]

In a similar case, a fifty-nine-year-old man underwent surgery for skin cancer and soon became confused and unable to stand without staggering. An alert neurologist determined the cause of his problems and started aggressive B$_{12}$ therapy. Within four weeks, the man could stand and walk again, and within eight weeks his memory and mental functions were back to normal.[9]

Unlike the surgeon who refused to evaluate our acquaintance for B$_{12}$ deficiency, even after he learned about the effects of N$_2$O, most doctors are too ethical to knowingly put their patients' lives in jeopardy. From a patient's point of view, however, it doesn't matter if a missed diagnosis of N$_2$O-caused damage stems from arrogance or ignorance, because the outcome is the same—pain, debility, paralysis, dementia, or even death.

The risks of GI surgery

We've described how surgeries involving N$_2$O can worsen an existing B$_{12}$ deficiency. Certain surgeries, however, can actually create a lifelong B$_{12}$ deficiency. This has nothing to do with anesthesia; instead, it happens because some operations can impair your digestive system's ability to absorb B$_{12}$. These include operations that involve removing part of the stomach or small intestine (and particularly a segment of the intestine called the terminal ileum), or gastric bypass surgeries to aid in weight loss.

If you undergo a gastrointestinal (GI) surgery, you don't need to worry, as long as your physician measures your B$_{12}$ and urinary MMA levels regularly and ensures that you receive B$_{12}$ injections or high-dose oral/sublingual B$_{12}$ if needed. But doctors often fail to do this, even in very high-risk patients. And many other doctors do test, but again make the mistake of assuming that the unreliable serum B$_{12}$ test alone can rule out a deficiency.

Thus, if you've had any type of gastrointestinal surgery, you'll need to take the initiative in protecting your health. If you aren't being monitored for B$_{12}$ problems, insist on testing, even if you have no symptoms. If your doctor says you've been tested, ask which tests were done. If you received only a serum B$_{12}$, insist on urinary MMA testing as well. If the tests come back normal, have them repeated yearly to ensure that a B$_{12}$ deficiency doesn't develop over time. Don't assume that your doctor is looking out for you, because it's not always the case (see sidebar).

An *Unheard Cry* for Help?

How many patients suffer devastating symptoms of B$_{12}$ deficiency after surgery because doctors either expose them to N$_2$O when they're already B$_{12}$-deficient, or fail to recognize and treat B$_{12}$-deficiency symptoms stemming from GI surgeries? Nobody knows. However, as an informal experiment, we asked a friend who does online research to quickly skim the Internet discussion groups and see if any possible cases turned up. Within fifteen minutes, she found a dozen cases that clearly sounded suspicious. Among the desperate comments of these patients are the following:

—"My surgeon never gave me B$_{12}$ after [gastric bypass] surgery. Eventually, after getting so sick that I could not walk any longer (and calling the doctor several times asking for help, but being told that I'll "get through it" and that it's "just natural to feel this way"), I was admitted to the hospital where they gave me what the doctor said was "triple the normal dose" of B$_{12}$." Sadly, this patient noted that he received no additional B$_{12}$ after this one dose, and he continues to suffer from worsening symptoms. He adds, "Now with a heavy mixture of Neurontin and Lortab from a neurologist who says that I have experienced nerve damage, I am barely able to go back to work or actually do anything besides sit there in tears."

—"I had general anesthesia during cataract surgery.... After the second eye was done, I became completely unable to get in and out of bed by myself. I was told it was due to general anesthesia and would go away in a few days. [But months later there is] no change, except maybe to get worse."

—"My husband has had an ileostomy for twelve years. Just within the past three years, he has begun experiencing some serious problems related to the nervous system. He now has a condition called trigeminal neuralgia, which is a dysfunction of the cranial nerve, causing excruciating pain in his face. In the last several months, he has been losing his grip in his hands and having difficulty with speech. Because of our limited insurance plan, he has been only able to see doctors who don't really know much about this and are just medicating him and pretty much telling him he'll have to live with these things."

—"Eight weeks ago I had a gallbladder attack and a few days later had laparoscopic surgery... within a day after the surgery, I started suffering from a persistent dizziness.... I've also had blurry vision, tingling and 'pins and needles' feelings in my extremities, chest pain [and] a 'wired but tired' feeling.... I've had an MRI, which came back normal. A blood panel showed no sign of anemia." *(Authors' note: As we explained earlier, a blood panel alone cannot diagnose B$_{12}$ deficiency accurately, and an MRI will not detect early damage.)* "...I've had many friends tell me that the anesthesia from the surgery could be the culprit. But both my doctor and the surgeon dismiss the notion."

—"I've had Crohn's [an inflammatory intestinal disease] for over twenty-five years; last four years have had increasing symptoms first in feet, now also in my hands. Had back surgery twice for stenosis of lumbar spine, then was re-diagnosed with peripheral neuropathy. Surgery once for Crohn's, removing terminal ileum. Have been tested a few times for B$_{12}$ deficiency, am told it reads normal. I take over-the-counter B$_{12}$ tablets, though I understand that's mainly a futile gesture. My neurologist wants to work me up to determine what kind of neuropathy, perhaps it's a type which is treatable, but my primary care doc won't even return my phone calls, is too busy defending the insurance company's bottom line."

Do any of these patients have B$_{12}$ deficiency resulting from their surgeries? It's very likely, given their symptom patterns. All are in desperate need of in-depth testing, and their cases suggest that victims of post-surgery B$_{12}$ deficiency aren't rare—just rarely identified.

Notes

1. McNeely, James K., Buczulinski, Bogdan, and Rosner, Diane R. Severe neurological impairment in an infant after nitrous oxide anesthesia. *Anesthesiology* (2000), 93:1549–50.

2. Holloway, Kathryn, and Alberico, Anthony. Postoperative myeloneuropathy:A preventable complication in patients with B$_{12}$ deficiency. *Journal of Neurosurgery* (May 1990), 72:732–6.

3. Marié, Rose-Marie, Le Biez, Eric, Busson, Philippe, Schaeffer, Stéphane, Boiteau, Lydia, Dupuy, Benoit, and Viader, Fausto. Nitrous oxide anesthesia-associated myelopathy. *Archives of Neurology* (March 2000), 57:380–2.

4. Hobbhahn, J. Are inhaled anaesthetics still toxic? educational paper, provided by the European Society of Anaesthesiologists (ESA), April 2000 http://www.euroanesthesia.org/pages/education/rc_Vienna/03rc1.HTM

5. Holloway, Kathryn, and Alberico, Anthony. Postoperative myeloneuropathy:A preventable complication in patients with B$_{12}$ deficiency. *Journal of Neurosurgery* (May 1990), 72:732–6.

6. Schilling, Robert. Is nitrous oxide a dangerous anesthetic for vitamin B$_{12}$-deficient subjects? *Journal of the American Medical Association* March 28, 1986, 255:1605–6.

7. Marié, Rose-Marie, Le Biez, Eric, Busson, Philippe, Schaeffer, Stéphane, Boiteau, Lydia, Dupuy, Benoit, and Viader, Fausto. Nitrous oxide anesthesia-associated myelopathy. *Archives of Neurology* March 2000, 57:380–2.

8. Hadzic, A., Glab, K., Sanborn, K., and Thys, D. Severe neurologic deficit after nitrous oxide anesthesia. *Anesthesiology* 1995, 83:863–6.

9. Flippo, Teresa, and Holder, Walter. Neurologic degeneration associated with nitrous oxide anesthesia in patients with vitamin B$_{12}$ deficiency. *Archives of Surgery* December 1993, 128:1391–1395.

Can't Conceive? How B_{12} Deficiency Contributes to Male and Female Infertility

"Vitamin B_{12} deficiency is associated with infertility.... Pregnancy may occur in the presence of B_{12} deficiency but may be associated with recurrent early fetal loss." —hematologist Michael Bennett, M.D.[1]

"A deficiency of B_{12} leads to reduced sperm counts and sperm motility." —Joseph Pizzorno, M.D., and Michael Murray, M.D.[2]

Millions of couples each year are thrilled to learn that their dream of starting a family is becoming a reality. But for one in eight couples who want children, the dream becomes a nightmare of sadness and frustration as months or even years pass, and the pregnancy tests keep saying "negative." For others, there is the terrible tragedy of miscarrying a baby—and the even greater tragedy of miscarrying time after time.

For infertile couples, life often becomes an endless round of expensive (and often unsuccessful) fertility treatments. For couples who conceive babies but suffer miscarriages, trying again to become pregnant can be frightening, turning what should be a happy life experience into an anxiety-ridden ordeal that often ends, once again, in failure.

There are dozens of common causes of male and female infertility, ranging from endometriosis, pelvic inflammatory disease, and polycystic ovary disease in women, to structural or hormonal problems in males, and to anti-sperm antibodies in either partner. But there is another risk factor for both male and female infertility that is often overlooked, even by infertility specialists. That problem is vitamin B$_{12}$ deficiency.

One miscarriage is sad enough, but the woman described by physician Michael Bennett had lost seven babies before birth. After years of suffering, she was lucky to find Dr. Bennett, a hematologist (a doctor specializing in blood abnormalities), who identified her severe B$_{12}$ deficiency. He treated her with injected B$_{12}$, and nine months later she delivered a healthy baby. Since then, she's given birth to two more children.[3]

The woman whose case Dr. Bennett reported was one of fourteen women he's seen over eleven years who suffered from infertility or recurrent miscarriages because of B$_{12}$ deficiency. Of these women, ten conceived successfully after receiving vitamin B$_{12}$ treatment, most within a matter of weeks. (The three remaining women were no longer trying to conceive at the time their deficiency was diagnosed.)

Bennett notes that many of these women had been evaluated by obstetricians and had undergone hormonal treatments, "but the vitamin B$_{12}$ deficiency was not recognized, and only much later were they sent for a hematologic consultation."

Married for seven years, the thirty-three-year-old woman kept hoping for a baby and wondering why she couldn't conceive. She also felt increasingly weak, had trouble walking, and noticed that she didn't remember things well.

Her doctors drew a blank, until one spotted signs of macrocytic anemia and referred her to a hematology clinic. There, doctors diagnosed her with B$_{12}$ deficiency and started her on injections of the vitamin.

Within three months, she felt vastly better mentally and she could walk normally again. Within six months, she became pregnant. Her long years of waiting for a child ended when she delivered a healthy baby girl.[4]

Other doctors have also reported successful pregnancies in once-infertile women following therapy for B$_{12}$ deficiency. Yet often, sadly, this deficiency is overlooked even by infertility specialists until women have undergone months or even years of unsuccessful treatment. As a result, many couples spend thousands of dollars, and they experience disappointment after disappointment, when treatment with B$_{12}$ injections might have solved their problem.

One group of London doctors, for instance, reported the case of a thirty-year-old woman with a history of infertility due in part to tubal disease. She underwent two attempts at *in vitro* fertilization, an expensive and time-consuming procedure, which both failed, with the second attempt producing far fewer oocytes (eggs) than the first. At a later visit to her doctor's office, where she complained about abnormal sensations in her hands, the doctor ordered a blood test that revealed low vitamin B$_{12}$ levels. The diagnosis: pernicious anemia. After treatment with injected B$_{12}$, she underwent another round of *in vitro* fertilization, this time producing a healthy number of eleven oocytes. However, she did not become pregnant, and the doctors say, "In retrospect, it may have been prudent to have waited for vitamin B$_{12}$ treatment to restore the endometrial function, before starting a further IVF cycle."

The doctors who report this case note that anovulation (a failure to release an egg during the monthly cycle) occurs in some women with B$_{12}$ deficiency due to pernicious anemia, and that B$_{12}$ deficiency also causes abnormalities of the cells of the reproductive tract (see Chapter 7) which may extend to the lining of the uterus. In addition, they note, B$_{12}$ deficiency is associated with abnormal estrogen levels that interfere with implantation of the fertilized egg.

Surprisingly, the doctors conclude, "We believe that the relation between vitamin B$_{12}$ deficiency and infertility needs more study before serum B$_{12}$ assays are to be included as a routine procedure in investigation of all infertile female patients to detect early cases of vitamin B$_{12}$ deficiency."[5] We disagree, because a serum B$_{12}$ test costs approximately sixty dollars, and the more accurate urinary MMA test costs as little as seventy dollars. Either expense pales in comparison to the thousands of dollars that couples spend on *in vitro* fertilization, a procedure which can fail if B$_{12}$ deficiency exists—and which might not even be necessary when patients with such a deficiency are properly treated.

Another thirty-two-year-old infertile woman whose case is reported in the medical literature underwent four rounds of artificial insemination without success, before her doctors detected both iron deficiency and vitamin B$_{12}$ deficiency. They began treatment with oral iron and injected vitamin B$_{12}$, and within two months, the woman became pregnant. She now has two healthy children, the second conceived without any need for fertility treatments.[6]

Researchers aren't yet sure why B$_{12}$ deficiency makes it difficult to conceive a baby, or to carry a baby to term. Dr. Bennett and his colleagues suggest that deficient B$_{12}$ levels interfere with ovulation or

---

B$_{12}$ Deficiency and Miscarriage: Far More Common than Doctors Think

A recurring theme in the medical literature is that B$_{12}$ deficiency is a fairly rare cause of miscarriage or stillbirth. The evidence, however, suggests otherwise.

One recent study, for instance, compared thirty-six women who'd suffered recurrent fetal loss to forty women who'd carried healthy babies to term. The researchers found that 31 percent of the women who'd lost several babies had high homocysteine levels. (Elevated homocysteine, as we noted in Chapter 5, is caused by low levels of folic acid, B$_{12}$, and/or vitamin B$_6$, and is easily treated with these vitamins.) Sixteen percent of the women who'd suffered recurrent fetal loss carried two copies of the MTHFR gene that causes abnormally high homocysteine levels, and three of the women had overt B$_{12}$ deficiency.[7]

---

normal cell division in the fertilized ovum, and that changes in the uterine lining due to B$_{12}$ deficiency prevent implantation. The high homocysteine levels that can result from poor B$_{12}$ status, they say, could cause fetal death by contributing to thrombosis (abnormal blood clotting), inadequate blood supply to the placenta, preeclampsia (which can lead to convulsions), premature separation of the placenta, or fetal growth retardation.

Whatever the reasons for the link between B$_{12}$ and infertility or miscarriage, Dr. Bennett and colleagues say the number of cases they've identified in their own practice "illustrates the importance of measuring B$_{12}$ levels... in every patient investigated for infertility or recurrent abortion." This is particularly critical, they say, now that women of childbearing age receive large amounts of folic acid from supplements or fortified foods.

Such testing will help many women to become pregnant, and in addition, it will protect many children against the devastating effects of B$_{12}$ deficiency in utero. As we've noted elsewhere, insufficient B$_{12}$ in the developing infant is linked to serious and potentially fatal problems, including neural tube defects (see Chapter 3) and neurological abnormalities that can lead to mental retardation or autism (see Chapter 6).

Male infertility and B$_{12}$ deficiency

In about 40 percent of cases, a couple's inability to conceive is due to male infertility. Here again, vitamin B$_{12}$ plays a significant role—and, again, that role is generally overlooked by doctors.

The link between male infertility and insufficient B$_{12}$ levels first became commonly known in the 1980s, when researchers reported a study in which 27 percent of men with sperm counts less than 20 million were able to increase these counts to more than 100 million after receiving 1,000 mcg per day of vitamin B$_{12}$.[8] This research was pursued by scientists in Japan, who published a series of clinical and laboratory studies showing B$_{12}$'s beneficial effects on sperm counts. Among their findings were the following:

- One research group administered high-dose oral B$_{12}$ to mice previously given a drug that lowered sperm counts. After ten weeks, they say, sperm count, sperm motility, motile sperm count, and percentage of "good" sperm were all increased in B$_{12}$-treated mice as compared to controls. "These results suggest that [B$_{12}$] enhanced the testicular function," they concluded, "resulting in an increased output of mature sperm."[9]
- In another study, 57 percent of men with low sperm counts showed increases in sperm number after receiving 6,000 mcg of B$_{12}$ per day.[10]
- A different research group tested the effects of B$_{12}$, Clomid (a fertility drug generally used to treat women, but also used in some cases to treat men), and B$_{12}$ plus Clomid on infertile men. They found that for infertile men with sperm counts higher than 10 million/ml, the combination of B$_{12}$ and Clomid increased sperm count in 80 percent of cases (and B$_{12}$ alone increased sperm count in more than 60 percent).[11] In another study, this group reported that when twenty-six infertile men were treated with B$_{12}$ at a fertility clinic, sperm

concentration increased in 38 percent of the men, total sperm counts increased in nearly 54 percent, sperm motility increased in 50 percent, and total motile sperm count increased in 50 percent.[12]

A newer study sheds light on the connection between B$_{12}$ and male fertility, by showing that low B$_{12}$ levels affect both gonadal and sperm health. Researchers who deprived rats of B$_{12}$ found that the rats exhibited atrophy of the seminiferous tubules (where sperm are produced), as well as poor development of sperm.[13]

There's evidence, too, that supplemental B$_{12}$ may also help men whose infertility stems from causes other than deficient B$_{12}$. Studies of rodents with testicular dysfunction induced by X-ray irradiation reveal that high-dose vitamin B$_{12}$ can increase the diameter of the seminiferous tubules and increase sperm counts.[14]

Infertility treatment: first things first

Americans spend millions of dollars each year on fertility drugs, artificial insemination, and *in vitro* fertilization. There is a place for these drugs and interventions, but only when simple, safe, inexpensive measures are exhausted.

High on the list of such measures, for men or women dealing with infertility issues, is getting tested for B$_{12}$ status. This testing must include a serum B$_{12}$ level, a urinaryMMA test, and a homocysteine test (see Chapter 10). These simple tests, if provided routinely to infertile couples, might spare thousands of men and women the suffering caused by infertility, miscarriages, and stillbirths.

Professor Ralph Gräsbeck, together with Olga Imerslund (noted discoverers of hereditary cubilin failure with cobalamin deficiency), describes how vitamin B$_{12}$ and folate deficiencies can cause infertility. Gräsbeck suggests that "Every case of infertility in primary health care should initially be managed by test treatment with micronutrients, before reproduction specialists are consulted."[15]

Notes

1.   Bennett, M. Vitamin B$_{12}$ deficiency, infertility and recurrent fetal loss. *Journal of Reproductive Medicine* 2001, 46(3):209–12.
2.   Pizzorno, J. and Murray, M. "Male Infertility," in *Textbook of Natural*

Medicine, Bastyr University, 1993 (online) http://www.healthy.net/library/books/textbook/Section6/MALEIN.PDF.

3. Bennett, M. Vitamin B$_{12}$ deficiency, infertility and recurrent fetal loss. *Journal of Reproductive Medicine* 2001, 46(3):209–12.

4. Menachem, Y., Cohen, A. M., and Mittelman, M. Cobalamin deficiency and infertility. *American Journal of Hematology* 1994, 46(2):152.

5. El-Nemr, A., Sabatini, L., Wilson, C., Lower, A. M., Al-Shawaf, T., and Grudzinska, J. G. Vitamin B$_{12}$ deficiency and IVF. *Journal of Obstetrics and Gynecology* 1998, 18(2):192–3.

6. Sanfilippo, J,. and Liu, Y. Vitamin B$_{12}$ deficiency and infertility: Report of a case. *International Journal of Fertility* 1991, 36(1):36–8.

7. Raziel, A., Kornberg, Y., Friedler, S., Schachter, M., Sela, B. A., and Ron-El, R. Hypercoagulable thrombophilic defects and hyperhomocysteinemia in patients with recurrent pregnancy loss. *American Journal of Reproductive Immunology* 2001, 45(2):65–71.

8. Sandler, B., and Faragher, B. Treatment of oligospermia with vitamin B$_{12}$. *Infertility* 1984, 7:133–8; cited in Pizzorno and Murray, "Male Infertility," in *Textbook of Natural Medicine*, Bastyr University, 1993 (online) http://www.healthy.net/library/books/textbook/Section6/MALEIN.PDF.

9. Oshio, S., Ozaki, S., Ohkawa, I., Tajima, T., Kaneko, S., and Mohri, H. Mecobalamin promotes mouse sperm maturation. *Andrologia* 1989, 21(2):167–73.

10. Kumamoto, Y., et al. Clinical efficacy of mecobalamin in treatment of oligospermia. Results of a double-blind comparative clinical study. *Acta Urologica Japan* 1988, 34:1109–32; cited in Pizzorno and Murray, "Male Infertility," in *Textbook of Natural Medicine*, Bastyr University, 1993 (online) http://www.healthy.net/library/books/textbook/Section6/MALEIN.PDF.

11. Isoyama, R., Baba, Y., Harada, H., Kawai, S., Shimizu, Y., Fujii, M., Fujisawa, S., Takihara, H., Koshido, Y., and Sakatoku, J. Clinical experience of methylcobalamin (CH3-B12)/clomiphene citrate combined treatment in male infertility. *Hinyokika Kiyo* 1986, 32(8):1177–83.

12. Isoyama, R., Kawai, S., Shimizu, Y., Harada, H., Takihara, H., Baba, Y., and Sakatoku, J. Clinical experience with methylcobalamin (CH3-B12) for male infertility. *Hinyokika Kiyo* 1984, 30(4):581–6.

13. Kawata, T., Tamiki, A., Tashiro, A., Suga, K., Kamioka, S., Yamada, K., Wada, M., Tanaka, N., Tadokoro, T., and Maekawa, A. Effect of vitamin B$_{12}$ deficiency on testicular tissue in rats fed by pair-feeding. *International Journal of Vitamin and Nutrition Research* 1997, 67(1):17–21.

14. Oshio, S., Yazaki, T., Umeda, T., Ozaki, S., Ohkawa, I., Tajima, T., Yamada, T., and Mohri, H. Effects of mecobalamin on testicular dysfunction induced by X ray irradiation in mice. *Nippon Yakurigaku Zasshi* 1991, 98(6):483–90.

15. Gräsbeck R. Infertility—folate, cobalamin and other micronutrients [evaluation]. Rondel 2002; 10. URL: www.rondellen.net.

10

Protecting Yourself: Are You at Risk for Vitamin B$_{12}$ Deficiency?

"I have been convinced all of my life that an informed patient is the best patient. My advice to people has always been, 'Take charge of your health.' Now it's more important than ever because, with managed care, no one else is." —C. Everett Koop, M.D., former surgeon general of the United States[1]

If you've read to this point, you're probably asking yourself: "Should I be worried?"

It's a smart question, because millions of people suffer from B$_{12}$ deficiency, and far too few ever get an accurate diagnosis. That's why you need to take matters into your own hands, in order to protect your health and your life. In this chapter, we'll tell you how to determine if you're one of the victims of this silent epidemic—and, if so, what you need to do.

Remember, as you read through this chapter, that B$_{12}$ deficiency is a "good news" diagnosis. That's because it's simple to treat, and if it's caught in time, your symptoms will vanish. Even if your B$_{12}$ deficiency is long-term, and not all of your symptoms are reversible, a correct diagnosis and proper treatment will help to prevent them from getting any worse. And, the treatment for this disorder costs only a few dollars a year, making it easy on your pocketbook.

So, if you suspect after reading this chapter that deficient B$_{12}$ levels could be playing a role in your medical problems, don't hesitate—find out!

Calculating Your Odds

B$_{12}$ deficiency isn't like the measles or a sprained ankle. There's no obvious symptom, like a red rash or a swollen joint, which allows you (or your doctor) to make an instant diagnosis. Instead, there are risk factors and symptom patterns that can strongly implicate deficient B$_{12}$ as a culprit. To know if you're at risk for B$_{12}$ deficiency, you need to recognize these risks and symptoms. If you spot them, your next step should be to call your doctor.

How can you tell if you're at risk? On the following pages, you'll find a checklist of the risk factors and symptoms most often associated with B$_{12}$ deficiency, along with a point score to assign to each of these. To make the checklist easier to use, we've divided it into categories. To determine your risk, add up your point score for all of the categories, and check it against the scoring chart at the end. If you are filling in the questionnaire for a loved one, simply answer as that person would.

Are You at Risk?

1. Neurological Symptoms

If you have any of the symptoms listed below, give yourself two points. If you have more than one of the symptoms listed below, give yourself another point for each additional symptom.

- Do you experience a "pins and needles" feeling or numbness in your feet, hands, legs, and/or arms?
- Have you been diagnosed with diabetic or peripheral neuropathy?
- Do you suffer from weakness in your arms and/or legs?
- Do you experience light-headedness or dizziness?
- Are you prone to falling or do you fall frequently?
- Have you or others noticed any unusual changes in your ability to move—for instance, do you walk clumsily, or with your feet wide apart, or have difficulty writing legibly?
- Have you noticed problems with your memory or thinking— for instance, increased difficulty in remembering names or dates, or more trouble in adding numbers, balancing your checkbook, or making change? Do you sometimes become

confused or disoriented? Do you suffer from memory problems or other symptoms of dementia?

- Do you have trouble knowing where various parts of your body are, if you aren't looking? (For instance, do you have trouble walking in the dark, when you can't see your feet?)
- Does your sense of touch, or your perception of pain, appear distorted?
- Has a doctor ever told you that you have muscular spasticity (lack of coordination and excessive muscle contraction)?
- Do you have a tremor?
- Do you suffer from urinary incontinence or impotence?

2. Psychiatric Symptoms

If you have any of the symptoms listed below, give yourself two points. If you have more than one of the symptoms listed below, give yourself another point for each additional symptom.

- Have you undergone any unusual personality changes—for instance, do your friends say that you're "not acting like yourself"—or do you find that you are more irritable than usual?
- Are you unusually apathetic or depressed, or have you ever been diagnosed with depression (including postpartum depression)? Have you ever had suicidal thoughts?
- Do you ever experience hallucinations or delusions?
- Do you ever exhibit violent behavior?
- Have you been diagnosed with any other form of psychosis or mental illness, including schizophrenia or bipolar disorder?
- Do you find yourself becoming more paranoid about other people's actions or intentions?

3. Hematologic Signs (Abnormalities of the blood cells)

If you have any of the signs listed below, give yourself two points. If you have more than one of the signs listed below, give yourself another point for each additional symptom.

- Has a doctor ever told you that you have abnormally small

red blood cells, an iron deficiency, or iron deficiency anemia?
- Has a doctor ever told you that you are anemic (low blood
count or low hemoglobin)? Do you have low platelets, or a
low white blood cell count?
- Has a doctor ever told you that your red blood cells are abnormally large (macrocytosis)?

4. Gastrointestinal Risk Factors

*If you have any of the risk factors listed below, give yourself
two points. If you have more than one of the risk factors
listed below, give yourself another point for each additional
symptom.*

- Have you been diagnosed with inflammation and/or wasting
of the stomach lining (gastric atrophy)?
- Have you been diagnosed as having low stomach acid?
- Do you suffer from gastritis?
- Do you suffer from ulcers?
- Have you been diagnosed with gastroesophageal reflux dis-
ease (GERD)?
- Do you have diverticulosis?
- Have you been diagnosed with precancerous gastrointestinal
growths or gastrointestinal cancer?
- Have you undergone a gastrointestinal resection (partial or
complete gastrectomy), undergone a gastric bypass surgery
for weight loss, or had either partial or complete removal of
your ileum (last part of the small intestine)?
- Have you been diagnosed with a malabsorption syndrome
(Crohn's disease, inflammatory bowel disease, irritable bowel
syndrome, or celiac disease [gluten enteropathy])?
- Do you have a family history of pernicious anemia (an autoimmune disease)?
- Have you been diagnosed with small bowel overgrowth?
- Have you been diagnosed with a tapeworm or other gastrointestinal parasite?

5. General Risk Factors

If you have any of the risk factors listed below, give yourself one point.

- Are you over the age of sixty?
- Do you have a thyroid disorder, or do you have an autoimmune disorder—for instance, lupus, insulin-dependent diabetes, rheumatoid arthritis, Hashimoto's thyroiditis, Graves' disease, Addison's disease, hypogammaglobulinemia, or a-gammaglobulinemia?
- Have you ever had cancer? Have you undergone chemotherapy, or undergone radiation therapy?
- Have you ever undergone surgery (including dental surgery) in which nitrous oxide was used?
- Do you abuse nitrous oxide as a recreational drug?
- Are you a vegan or vegetarian?
- Are you an alcoholic?
- Are you taking any of the following medications: H-2 blockers (Pepcid, Zantac, Tagamet, Axid), potassium chloride (K-dur), Glucophage, Glucovance, proton pump inhibitors (Nexium, Prevacid, Prilosec, Protonix), birth control pills, colchicine, Questran, neomycin, or drugs that treat tuberculosis?

6. Other Signs/Symptoms often Associated with B$_{12}$ Deficiency

If you have any of the signs or symptoms listed below, give yourself one point.

- Do you suffer from fatigue, lack of energy, or weakness?
- Do you suffer from generalized weakness?
- Have you experienced a loss of weight or loss of appetite?
- Do you suffer from chest pain, or from shortness of breath with exertion (e.g., walking from your bed to the toilet or to your kitchen)?
- Do you have areas of skin hypopigmentation (unusually light spots), or have you been diagnosed with vitiligo?
- Are you unusually pale, or do you have a lemon-yellow skin color?

- Do you have a sore, inflamed, or "beefy red" tongue?
- Do you suffer from tinnitus (ringing in the ears)?
- If you are female, has a doctor ever told you that your Pap smear showed abnormal cells (cervical dysplasia)?
- Do you suffer from infertility?

To Calculate Your Score:

Add the points in every category. Your score is:
Low Risk: with less than 3 points
Moderate Risk: with 3 to 6 points
High Risk: if your points are greater than 6

What should you do now?

If you scored in the low-risk range, and you do not have any of the medical conditions listed in the section following this one, your B$_{12}$ levels are probably fine. Remember, however, that as you age, your B$_{12}$ levels may drop—meaning that a healthy level today won't guarantee that you're safe two years from now—so be aware of the symptoms and risk factors we've described, and have your B$_{12}$ and MMA levels checked if you develop any of them.

If you scored in the moderate-risk range and are not experiencing any symptoms, wait until your next doctor's appointment and then insist on having a urinary MMA test. If you're actively suffering from any symptoms that could be caused by insufficient B$_{12}$, however, make an appointment as soon as possible. If B$_{12}$ deficiency is indeed the culprit, catching it early may lead to a complete remission of symptoms.

If you scored in the high-risk range, there is no time to waste: Call your doctor, and get the earliest appointment possible. Once you're there, make sure you receive urinary MMA testing (discussed later in this chapter). If your doctor is skeptical or resistant, be assertive—and, if necessary, find another doctor.

Are there specific medical conditions that put me at risk?

Regardless of your score on this questionnaire, we believe that if you currently suffer from, or have suffered from, any of the following conditions, you need to be tested for B$_{12}$ deficiency:

- dementia/Alzheimer's disease
- multiple sclerosis
- autism
- any neurologic disorder
- any psychiatric disorder
- peripheral neuropathy (related to diabetes or other disorders)
- AIDS or AIDS dementia complex
- optic neuritis
- hyperhomocysteinemia
- congestive heart failure
- insulin-dependent diabetes mellitus (IDDM) (also known as Type I diabetes)
- fibromyalgia
- vertigo

You also need to be tested if you are undergoing or have undergone hemodialysis, suffer from chronic pain, or have an occlusive vascular disorder—transient ischemic attacks (TIAs or mini-strokes), cerebrovascular accident (CVA or stroke), pulmonary embolism (blood clot in the lung), myocardial infarction (heart attack), coronary artery disease, or deep vein thrombosis. People with iron deficiency anemia, radiculopathy (nerve irritation in an arm or leg, from a back or neck disorder or from surgery), a history of alcoholism, or the blood disorders polycythemia or thrombocytopenia should also be tested. Vitamin B$_{12}$ deficiency can cause signs and symptoms that mimic or hide behind many of these diseases.

What tests should I have?

If you score in the moderate-risk or high-risk range, your doctor needs to order a sensitive test that detects B$_{12}$ deficiency at the tissue or cellular level. This test is a measurement of your urinary methylmalonic acid (MMA) level. This is the key test that will tell you if you are B$_{12}$-deficient, and it must be performed in order to conclusively diagnose or rule out B$_{12}$ deficiency.

We recommend the urinary MMA, a non-invasive test that will show if there is elevated MMA in the urine. This is an indication of tissue or cellular B$_{12}$ deficiency, because it is directly related to a B$_{12}$-dependent metabolic pathway. When that pathway is interrupted due to insufficient B$_{12}$, MMA levels in the urine rise. The urine MMA is a very sensitive and accurate test, and it can be adjusted for urine dilution, which is important if you suffer from kidney (renal) disease or dehydration.

Another test, the serum B$_{12}$ test, is the test doctors typically use to measure B$_{12}$ levels. This is a useful test, but for some people it is not the most accurate measure of B$_{12}$ status. In fact, while it may seem strange, it's possible to have a normal or even high serum B$_{12}$ level and be dangerously deficient in B$_{12}$ (see Chapter 11).

Throughout this book, we also recommend a third test called serum homocysteine (Hcy). This test isn't specific for B$_{12}$ deficiency, because a high Hcy can indicate low B$_{12}$, B$_{6}$, or folic acid levels, as well as other medical conditions, such as renal failure or untreated hypothyroidism. In addition, elevated Hcy can stem from the use of certain medications. However, the Hcy is a valuable adjunctive screening tool that can help you lower your risk of cardiovascular disease (see Chapter 5), and it can help confirm a diagnosis of B$_{12}$ deficiency because Hcy is almost always elevated when B$_{12}$ is dangerously low.

While the Hcy test is useful, it can also be misused. As we discussed earlier, many doctors make the mistake of detecting high homocysteine levels and immediately start folic acid treatment, without checking to determine if the problem stems instead from a deficiency of vitamin B$_{12}$. It's crucial, if your Hcy result is high, to find out if your high homocysteine is caused by deficient B$_{12}$ levels, because taking folic acid won't help if the root cause is a B$_{12}$ deficiency—and, even worse, the folic acid will mask the traditional blood cell changes of B$_{12}$ deficiency, while allowing the neurologic damage to continue and progress. So remember our rule: The Hcy test must be part of a total "package," including urinary MMA and serum B$_{12}$ testing.

If you or a family member has symptoms that are diagnosed as multiple sclerosis, a childhood developmental disability, autism, or other conditions we've covered in separate chapters, check these chapters for additional tests that we recommend. Also, if you prove to be B$_{12}$-deficient, your doctor should run further tests to see if you suffer from pernicious anemia, an autoimmune disease that causes B$_{12}$ deficiency, or another malabsorption disorder.

What about treatment?

In our opinion, B$_{12}$ injections are preferable to oral B$_{12}$ in many cases, and *they are absolutely necessary when neurological symptoms are present.* This is an area of controversy, but we've personally seen cases where oral B$_{12}$ simply didn't work, and such cases are reported in the literature as well.

Many doctors will argue that the literature indicates—although it does not prove—that oral B$_{12}$ is adequate in most cases (see Chapter 11 for an extensive discussion of this topic). Our philosophy is simply this: Given that monthly shots of B$_{12}$ are virtually painless thanks to new microfine needles, and given the multiple ways (see Chapter 1) in which the B$_{12}$ pathway can be disrupted between your mouth and your bloodstream, why take a chance?

In addition, if you're counting pennies, the shots are cheaper than the pills if you inject yourself or have a family member administer the injections for you. Shots are also the safest route if you're dealing with a B$_{12}$-deficient loved one who is forgetful or non-compliant, and thus likely to skip oral doses. Tens of thousands of diabetics can testify—as can one of the coauthors of this book, who self-administers her B$_{12}$ shots each month—that the shots take only seconds to prepare and are simple to administer after the first time or two.

If you aren't sure if you can handle self-administering monthly shots, ask your doctor for a prescription and a little training, and give it a try for a month or two. We can just about guarantee that you'll find self-injections easier and more convenient than taking B$_{12}$ pills every day—and if not, you can always have your doctor's staff administer the shots, or have a family member trained to give them to you.

A *Final Word about* Oral B$_{12}$

We don't dismiss the use of oral B$_{12}$ supplements entirely, because recent studies do look promising. If you and your doctor agree on oral B$_{12}$, we recommend a high dose (1,000 mcg per day) in sublingual (under the tongue) form. You should switch to an oral formula only after you've received initial shots to get your B$_{12}$ stores back to normal, and you should have yearly urinary MMA tests to make sure the oral formula is working for you.

Don't quit!

A few causes of B$_{12}$ deficiency are temporary. Many, however, are permanent, and taking extra B$_{12}$ for a few weeks or months won't solve the problem. If you have one of these conditions, you'll need to take supplemental B$_{12}$ for life, and it's both your responsibility and your doctor's to make sure that there's no break in your treatment.

Sometimes doctors order serum B$_{12}$ tests for patients who've undergone long-term B$_{12}$ treatment, in order to demonstrate to these patients that they're not deficient—or even to convince them that they never suffered from a deficiency in the first place. This is misguided, because people who've been correctly treated for B$_{12}$ deficiency will have adequate serum B$_{12}$ levels, and these levels will stay adequate for months to years when treatment is stopped. Eventually, however, the deficiency will return—and, with it, the risk of debilitating symptoms, or even death.

In other cases, problems arise when patients switch to new doctors who aren't knowledgeable about B$_{12}$ deficiency. We recommend that patients who receive a diagnosis of B$_{12}$ deficiency obtain their test results and medical records, and give copies of these papers to any new doctors. A physician who's skeptical about your assertion that you're B$_{12}$-deficient is likely to be more accepting if you have the documentation to prove it. Again, however, this is a time to be assertive. If you know you're B$_{12}$-deficient, and a doctor says, "You don't need treatment for that any more," don't be afraid to speak up. Insist on treatment, and if you don't get it, find a more knowledgeable doctor.

Of course, as medical professionals, we're all too aware that this is easier said than done. As physician Charles Inlander points out in *Medicine on Trial*, "Doctors over recent generations have established the ground rules for patient behavior, especially regarding the patient's relationship to (and critique of) the doctor. Many of us are taught (or intuit) that it is not good form to play too active a role, never mind a contentious one. Questions to doctors should be polite and deferential, acknowledging their superior knowledge and the wisdom of experience. If we are irritated with the doctor's demeanor in any way or left with any uneasy feeling that something is not right in the care being given, we might save our gripes for relatives or friends."

Unfortunately, when it comes to B$_{12}$ deficiency, this politeness can be fatal. In our own practices, we've seen dozens of people who were diagnosed as B$_{12}$-deficient at some point in their lives but later allowed doctors to discontinue their treatment. Several paid a high price for this lack of assertiveness, because they now have permanent neurological damage or dementia.

Conversely, we know of patients with B$_{12}$ deficiency who are alive and well today only because they, or an assertive family member, insisted—sometimes in the face of significant resistance—on proper diagnosis and treatment.

Bill, an active seventy-seven-year-old retired engineer, had a history of pernicious anemia, diagnosed fifteen years earlier. Not long ago, Bill suffered a heart attack, and tests indicated that he needed a heart valve replacement. At the time, he was also suffering from severe iron-deficiency anemia. Bill's doctors suspected that the anemia stemmed from occult gastrointestinal bleeding, but they could find no evidence of this, so they simply gave him two units of blood to improve his anemia.

A few months later, Bill underwent successful surgery. After the operation, however, he began experiencing hand tremors, light-headedness, extreme weakness, and fatigue. As the weeks passed, he became increasingly weak and eventually could no longer walk. He became very anemic again, and required multiple blood transfusions. His surgeon, diagnosing Bill as iron-deficient because his red blood cells were very small, told Bill to take iron supplements.

The iron supplements didn't help, and Bill's condition continued to worsen. Bill's cardiologist, informed of his patient's decline, had him admitted to the emergency department, and Bill's nephew Michael, who happens to be a nurse at the same hospital, accompanied him there. Michael informed the ER doctor that Bill had pernicious anemia, and that he hadn't received a B$_{12}$ injection for at least four months. (Bill had been told by his family doctor prior to surgery that he didn't need the B$_{12}$ shots, and that they would interfere with his new heart medications— both untrue statements.)

Despite Michael's input, the ER doctor, and the other admitting physicians who cared for Bill during his hospital stay, did not order any B$_{12}$ testing or provide any treatment for Bill's symptoms. Michael called Bill's cardiologist, cardiovascular surgeon, internist, and general practitioner, but none would agree to investigate Bill for B$_{12}$ deficiency. In the course of his calls, Michael learned that the general practitioner treating

Bill's pernicious anemia had been administering B$_{12}$ shots only every three to four months, rather than monthly—thus setting the stage for Bill's postsurgical B$_{12}$ crisis.

When transfusions failed to help Bill, the cardiothoracic surgeon— persuaded in large part by Michael's determined advocacy—called in a hematologist (a specialist in blood disorders). While Bill's recent blood transfusions skewed his test results, as did his earlier pre-surgery transfusions, the doctor recognized Bill's clear-cut symptoms of deficiency and immediately began B$_{12}$ injections. By the third injection, Bill was remarkably improved, and he was soon discharged home. He could stand again, and his tremor, weakness, fatigue, and unsteadiness were dramatically reduced.

It took weeks, and a series of B$_{12}$ shots, for Bill to completely regain his strength, but his story has a happy ending: He's now fully recovered and back to enjoying life. The credit for his recovery belongs in large part to his nephew, who refused to take "no" for an answer when it came to his uncle's need for proper treatment.

Spread the word!

It's not unusual for B$_{12}$ deficiency to run in families, so if you're diagnosed with this disorder, let your relatives know. When the authors of this book urged other family members to have their B$_{12}$ levels checked, they uncovered several cases of B$_{12}$ deficiency which were causing symptoms ranging from dizziness, to tremor, to autistic behavior.

At first, your family members may tease you about your "over-zealousness" in educating them about the dangers of B$_{12}$ deficiency. (We can sympathize, because it's happened to us!) But if your generosity in sharing your new knowledge leads to a diagnosis for another family member, that teasing will quickly turn to gratitude. It may also lead to a cure for your relatives' troubling or life-threatening medical symptoms—and that's one of the greatest gifts you can give your loved ones.

Notes

1. Dr. Koop's remarks were made in an interview in the *Reformed Quarterly* (newsletter of the Reformed Theological Seminary), Winter 1998.

11

Information for Physicians

"Vitamin B$_{12}$ deficiency affects about one quarter of the U.S. population and is more common in the elderly and in adults with several predisposing conditions.... Health-care professionals need to recognize that vitamin B$_{12}$ deficiency is often undetected and can lead to devastating and irreversible complications. Early treatment is effective and prevents disability from hematologic or neuropsychiatric complications, or both."
—T. S. Dharmarajan, M.D., and Edward P. Norkus, Ph.D., in *Postgraduate Medicine*[1]

In the emergency department, we never know who will come through our doors next. On a typical shift our patients could include a confused elderly woman, a man complaining of chest pains, a young woman with puzzling neurological symptoms, a elderly man with a hip fracture, a pregnant woman suffering a miscarriage, a young man in the grip of an acute episode of paranoia, a depressed and suicidal patient, a stroke victim, an AIDS patient or diabetic crippled by neuropathy, or a child whose diagnosis is listed as "failure to thrive."

As we look over these patients' records, we see the obvious battery of tests—X rays, blood tests, psychiatric evaluations, EKGs, MRIs, CT scans. What we don't see, however, is evidence that a significant percentage of the patients who present with possible signs and symptoms of B$_{12}$ deficiency—including all of the patients we just described above—have been tested for this common, simple-to-treat, and potentially deadly problem.

Obviously, only a minority of the patients we treat have symptoms caused by deficient B$_{12}$. However, this problem affects as much as 25 percent of the population,[2] causing a remarkable array of debilitating and dangerous medical problems. Yet many physicians, including those who treat many older patients, will rarely or never diagnose a case of B_{12} deficiency.

Why? One reason is that physicians think of B_{12} deficiency only as a hematologic disorder. In reality, however, it damages the brain, spinal cord, peripheral nerves, and the nerves of the eye, often well before blood abnormalities appear. Thus, doctors who think of B_{12} deficiency only in the context of anemia will miss the majority of cases that pass through their offices. Physicians must become aware that *macrocytic anemia is often a late sign of vitamin B_{12} deficiency, frequently occurring long after potentially irreversible neurological damage has taken place.*

Another reason for the high rate of missed diagnoses is that B_{12} deficiency is a master mimic, masquerading as a wide variety of medical problems. It can present as dementia, psychosis, depression, vertigo, tremor, neuropathy, recurrent miscarriage, infertility, unexplained vision loss, fatigue, dizziness, or a daunting range of other symptoms. In infants and young children, it can present as conditions ranging from autistic-like disorders or mental retardation, to loss of appetite and "failure to thrive," to stroke. Patients with B_{12} deficiency may be asymptomatic, have few or subtle signs, or present with a wide variety of overt signs and symptoms that are easy to blame on preexisting diseases.

There is a historical reason, too, for doctors' failure to diagnose B_{12} deficiency. Many physicians remember the days when thousands of patients got B_{12} shots whether they needed them or not, and their justified scorn for this practice leads them to overreact by making the opposite mistake: failing to realize that B_{12} deficiency is, indeed, a real, common, and serious medical condition.

Even when physicians do consider B_{12} deficiency as a diagnostic possibility, they tend to order only a serum B_{12} test, which fails to reveal many cases of B_{12} deficiency. Serum B_{12} levels can be normal or even high in deficient patients—and, adding to the problem, the cutoff for "normal" serum B_{12} in the United States is considered by many experts to be far too low. There is a far more accurate test to determine B_{12} status (urinary methylmalonic acid), which we'll describe later in this chapter, but most doctors don't order it because they don't know what it is—or even that it exists. Even doctors who are aware of the test often aren't aware of its availability, or the need for tests more sensitive than serum B_{12}.

The combined result of these many factors is that millions of patients, both young and old, suffer because their physicians miss an easy diagnosis.

B$_{12}$'s crucial roles

Very few doctors are aware of the full range of problems that can stem from B$_{12}$ deficiency, and we frequently encounter skepticism when we tell physicians that their patients' low B$_{12}$ levels could be responsible for symptoms as diverse as dementia, heart disease, muscle weakness, and infertility. But deficient B$_{12}$ levels can indeed affect almost every system of the body, because cobalamin plays an integral role in a wide range of neurologic, hematologic, immunologic, metabolic, vascular, and reproductive functions including the following:

- the division of all cells
- numerous enzymatic reactions
- the synthesis of nucleic acids, the transmethylation of amino acids, and the metabolism of carbohydrates and fatty acids.
- maintenance of a healthy nervous system, because it maintains the myelin surrounding the central and peripheral nervous systems
- the proper function of folic acid, because it allows folic acid to assist in converting the amino acid homocysteine (Hcy) into the essential amino acid methionine. If vitamin B$_{12}$ is not present, folic acid becomes "trapped" and cannot function properly, leading to dangerously elevated levels of toxic homocysteine*

Because B$_{12}$ deficiency severely impairs many systems in the body, and because it is so easily treated, doctors should make it a point to routinely identify and treat its victims. This is particularly crucial now, as the "Baby Boomer" generation ages into its senior years—the years of highest risk for B$_{12}$-deficiency-related problems.

B$_{12}$ metabolism: a complex pathway

In its natural state, cobalamin occurs only in animal products. Unlike other vitamins, this large molecule must undergo several major steps

---

*When folic acid "trapping" occurs, Hcy is not converted into methionine, and Hcy levels begin to rise. The accumulation of Hcy in the blood is toxic to blood vessels, causing plaque formation which leads to occlusive vascular disorders such as coronary artery disease (CAD), myocardial infarctions (MI), cerebral vascular accidents (CVA), transient ischemic attacks (TIA), deep vein thromboses (DVT), and carotid and renal artery stenosis.

How Common Is B$_{12}$ Deficiency?

Coauthor Jeffrey Stuart, D.O., recently conducted a retrospective study of all emergency department patients for whom he personally had ordered B$_{12}$ levels, after observing possible risk factors for B$_{12}$ deficiency. (See appendices O and P.)

Dr. Stuart calculated the number of patients found to be B$_{12}$ deficient (Cbl level<180pg/ml) as well as those with levels between 180 and 211 pg/ml., and those in the indeterminate range of 212–350pg/ml. (He included the last range because hematology experts report that a significant number of patients in this range are deficient, and they recommend that these patients be screened using the more sensitive urinary MMA and plasma Hcy.[3] Some experts even advocate screening patients whose cobalamin levels are below 400pg/ml.[4])

The analysis included 302 patients. Of these, twenty-four (7.9 percent) were found to be overtly deficient, with levels of less than 180pg/ml. An additional sixteen (5.3 percent) patients were in the range of 180-211pg/ml, putting them at greatly elevated risk for deficiency. Finally, the 212-350pg/ml range included ninety-one (30.1 percent) patients who warranted further testing. Thus, a total of 131 patients, or 43.3 percent of the total, had B$_{12}$ levels less than 350pg/ml. Notably, of this group, 30 percent were less than sixty years of age.

These findings are consistent with other studies showing that 15 to 20 percent of seniors are B$_{12}$-deficient, and that as many as 40 percent of hospitalized elderly patients have low or borderline serum B$_{12}$ levels.[5] Additionally, as we note in Chapter 1, more than 80 percent of long-term vegans who do not supplement their diets correctly, and over 50 percent of long-term vegetarians, show clear evidence of B$_{12}$ deficiency.[6,7] Additional alarming evidence comes from the large-scale Framingham study, one of the most prestigious studies of all time, which found that nearly 40 percent of participants between the ages of twenty-six and eighty-three had plasma B$_{12}$ levels in the low-normal range—a level at which some people begin experiencing neurological symptoms.[8]

in the digestion process for its proper absorption, and a breakdown can occur at any of the following stages:

- In the stomach, vitamin B_{12} is released from its protein-bound state by pepsin. This step requires the acidic environment of a healthy stomach producing hydrochloric acid.
- The stomach's parietal cells also secrete intrinsic factor, which is required for B_{12} absorption.
- Once vitamin B_{12} is freed from its protein-bound state, it connects to salivary vitamin B_{12} receptors, called cobalo-philins, or R-binders.
- These complexes are further broken down in the duodenum by pancreatic proteases, which allow the released vitamin B_{12} to attach to intrinsic factor.
- When all of these steps are completed, the vitamin B_{12}-intrinsic factor complex is transported to the ileum. This complex adheres to receptors on the ileal cells and penetrates the mucosal wall.
- A plasma protein, transcobalamin II, carries vitamin B_{12} to the various cells of the body, and then transports the excess to the liver for storage.

The metabolism of B_{12} is a complex and easily disrupted process, and a variety of problems—genetic, digestive, metabolic, dietary, pharmaceutical, autoimmune—can stop it in its tracks. This explains why cobalamin deficiency is so widespread, despite the ready availability of this vitamin in a typical diet.

Who is at highest risk?

If you're a physician who treats adult patients—no matter what your specialty—the odds are that at least one of the patients you see this week will be at least moderately B_{12}-deficient. Even if you treat children or teens, your patients almost undoubtedly include some at risk for dangerously low B_{12}.

B_{12} deficiency can strike anyone, at any age, but some patients are at far greater risk than others. The majority of cases of B_{12} deficiency stem from malabsorption disorders (see Chapter 2), and seniors are at highest risk because 30 to 40 percent of them have atrophic gastritis.

This condition drastically decreases levels of the stomach acid needed to free B$_{12}$ from animal proteins, which is necessary so that it can be absorbed. However, malabsorption problems are also common in people of any age who have the following medical conditions (see Appendix A):

- Crohn's disease, blind loop syndrome, celiac disease, or other digestive disorders
- a history of gastrointestinal surgeries (including surgery for weight loss)
- a history of radiation treatment for GI or pelvic cancers

The second most common cause of B$_{12}$ deficiency is pernicious anemia (PA), in which an autoimmune process destroys the cells that produce intrinsic factor. PA can occur at any stage of life (one of the authors of this book was in her early twenties when she was diagnosed), but it is typically thought to develop in middle age or later. Although many doctors think of PA as a "northern European disease," recent studies show that it affects all ethnic groups. Genes play a strong role in PA, and immediate relatives of people with pernicious anemia have nearly twenty times the normal risk of developing the condition.[9]

A diet low in B$_{12}$ can also cause deficiency, and it frequently does so even in people with no other risk factors. In fact, one risk group for B$_{12}$ deficiency, largely overlooked by doctors, consists of health-conscious vegans and vegetarians. Many of these people fail to take the proper amount of supplemental B$_{12}$; a number of others take spirulina or tempeh, supplements that are touted as being high in B$_{12}$ but actually contain B$_{12}$ analogues that block the absorption of cobalamin and cause falsely normal serum B$_{12}$ levels on testing. Unless they are knowledgeable about nutrition, vegans and vegetarians can easily become deficient—as can infants who are nursed by B$_{12}$-deficient vegan or vegetarian mothers. In these infants, B$_{12}$ deficiency can manifest as motor problems, retardation, loss of language and social skills, or failure to thrive.

Infants also can develop B$_{12}$ deficiency if their mothers have undiagnosed pernicious anemia, particularly if the mothers breast-feed. In addition, some children suffer from inherited forms of B$_{12}$ deficiency, which often manifest early in life and can rapidly become fatal (see Chapter 12). It is important to determine which genetic error is present in order to treat a patient properly. (For instance, orotic aciduria is a genetic disorder of pyrimidine metabolism and patients present with megaloblastic anemia. This disorder does not respond to treatment with B_{12} or folic acid, but is treated with oral uridine.) Immediate treatment for any inborn error needs to be started to prevent permanent mental retardation and/or death.

Inherited defects are usually, but not always, obvious during infancy. Some are not apparent until early childhood, when they can take the form of developmental delays and can be mistaken for autism (see chapters 6 and 12). The problems of children with B_{12} deficiency due to genetic defects are often exacerbated by other insults that reduce B_{12} stores, such as nitrous oxide exposure, leaky gut syndrome, celiac disease, small bowel overgrowth, or even immunizations containing mercury.

Surgical patients are another group at high risk of suffering debility due to B_{12} deficiency. Nitrous oxide, a commonly used anesthetic, inactivates methylcobalamin by inducing irreversible oxidation on the cobalt atom of vitamin B_{12}. This can cripple or kill patients who go into the operating room with low B_{12} stores—particularly if they undergo surgical procedures requiring several hours of nitrous oxide exposure. In one report, researchers found that the urinary MMA in one patient rose to 314 mcg/ml creatinine (normal is less than 3.8) after nitrous oxide exposure for eighty minutes.[10] Because of the absence of preoperative B_{12}/urinaryMMA testing and the high prevalence of B_{12} deficiency, this problem is far more common than recognized. Doctors often fail to diagnose postsurgical B_{12} deficiency, assuming that patients' weakness, paralysis, or other symptoms are unfortunate but unavoidable side effects of their surgeries. When patients are elderly, surgeons may tend to blame age, rather than considering B_{12} deficiency. Some physicians, aware of nitrous oxide's effects, administer B_{12} shots prior to operations; however, this does not adequately protect patients who should receive a thorough screening before undergoing surgery, so that they can receive appropriate long-term care if they prove to be B_{12}-deficient.

Dental patients can also become B_{12}-deficient after long procedures using nitrous oxide, and several cases involving dentists and dental assistants have been reported in the medical literature.[11] Recreational users of nitrous oxide, a popular drug of abuse, can develop neurological problems and florid mental symptoms due to B_{12} depletion, and physicians should suspect this problem in any teen or young adult patient who develops MS-like symptoms, numbness, weakness, visual disturbance, depression, psychosis, or other mental or neurological problems.

A number of common prescription drugs, too, can deplete B$_{12}$ stores, particularly in older patients. Among the most common culprits are metformin (Glucophage), antacids, H-2 blockers, proton pump inhibitors, potassium chloride, colchicine, neomycin, and Questran. (See Appendix A for a more complete list.) In young and middle-aged women, birth control pills are a common culprit.

Sensitive adjunctive tests that aid in diagnosis

As we noted earlier, the standard serum B$_{12}$ test fails to identify many patients with low cobalamin levels. For example, patients with underlying liver disease, alcoholism, myeloproliferative disorders, lymphoma, or intestinal bacterial overgrowth often have falsely elevated serum B$_{12}$ levels. Fortunately, adjunctive tests that aid in the diagnosis of B$_{12}$ deficiency are available. These include tests for urine and serum methylmalonic acid (MMA) and plasma homocysteine (Hcy), two metabolites that are biochemical markers of B$_{12}$-dependent enzyme activity. (Homocysteine is often elevated in vitamin B$_{12}$ deficiency, but it also is elevated in untreated hypothyroidism, folic acid deficiency, vitamin B$_6$ deficiency, and renal insufficiency.**)

Because high levels of MMA and Hcy indicate B$_{12}$ deficiency at the tissue level, these tests can identify patients with a deficiency when serum B$_{12}$ levels are low or borderline, or even when they fall within the normal range. It is important to note, by the way, that these are not new tests; the urinary MMA has been available for twenty years and is highly recommended by leading authorities.

** While it's expected for MMA and Hcy levels to be elevated in dialysis patients and patients with renal insufficiency, nephrologists are now reporting that dialysis patients' MMA and Hcy levels can be lowered considerably by giving them injectable or IV methylcobalamin or hydroxocobalamin. This is of great interest, because renal patients are at high risk for thrombotic events and lowering Hcy may dramatically decrease that risk. In our opinion, continued research is needed to determine what percentage of patients with renal insufficiency also suffer from B$_{12}$ deficiency that is not diagnosed because of the overlap of symptoms and the fact that high MMA and Hcy levels are simply expected in these cases. A missed diagnosis of B$_{12}$ deficiency can drastically decrease the quality of life of patients already dealing with renal insufficiency/failure, by adding anemia, neuropathy, depression, fatigue, weakness, apathy, hyperhomocysteinemia, impaired balance, and tremors to the list of problems with which they must contend.

We strongly believe that the urinary MMA/creatinine ratio test is superior to other tests used to identify or rule out vitamin B_{12} deficiency, because other tests can give false-positive or false-negative results, while the urinary MMA/creatinine ratio test does not. The chart on pages 166 and 167 details the relative merits and drawbacks of each form of testing.

After a thorough review of the medical literature pertaining to the serum MMA and the urinary MMA/creatinine ratio tests, we firmly believe that the urinary MMA is preferable, particularly for elderly patients, or those with renal disease. The highly accurate urinary MMA, which is consistent regardless of changes in patients' medical status, helps to prevent under-or over-treatment. The urinary MMA is the only MMA test validated for screening senior populations, and clinicians can be confident that the results are accurate without having to simultaneously order the serum creatinine and CBC tests needed to correctly interpret the results of a serum MMA. In the emergency department setting, the urinary MMA is the only appropriate form of MMA testing, because of its accuracy regardless of hydration or renal status and the fact that it does not require a twelve-hour fast.***

Which of your patients should receive MMA testing, as well as other tests for B_{12} deficiency? After years of clinical experience and research, as well as an extensive review of the literature, we have developed the Cobalamin Deficiency Criteria List (CDCL) as a screening tool for doctors and other health-care providers (see Appendix M). The CDCL's point system allows physicians to estimate a patient's relative risk of B_{12} deficiency, defined as the Cobalamin Deficiency Risk (CDR) Score.

We recommend obtaining a serum B_{12} and urinary MMA for any patient whose CDR Score falls in the moderate-risk or high-risk categories. Patients with suspected multiple sclerosis or autism also need the serum unsaturated B_{12}-binding capacity test, and plasma homocysteine.

These tests are relatively inexpensive and will be reimbursed when

---

*** The urinary MMA/creatinine ratio test is readily available from the Norman Clinical Laboratory (2005 cost $70, www.b12.com), or the Mayo Clinic Laboratory (2005 cost $203.40). The test can detect B_{12} deficiency in approximately one hour, using a single urine specimen. It is important to find a laboratory that uses the GC/MS technique to identify MMA in the urine, such as the two laboratories listed above. Older methodology can lead to erroneous results, sometimes with devastating consequences—see the story of Patricia Stallings in Chapter 6.

Serum Vitamin B$_{12}$

1. Cost-effective when used in conjunction with the more accurate urinary MMA test. Not sufficient when used alone, because of its high degree of inaccuracy (see points 2 and 3 below).

2. Can give false-negative results (elevated serum B$_{12}$ levels in the presence of deficiency) in patients with the following conditions:

—active liver disease (hepatitis, alcoholism)
—transcobalamin II deficiency
—intestinal bacterial overgrowth
—myeloproliferative disorders
    —polycythemia vera
    —chronic myelogenous leukemia
    —acute promyelocytic leukemia
—chloral hydrate medication
—lymphoma

3. Can give false-positive results (low serum B$_{12}$ levels in the absence of deficiency) in patients with the following conditions:

—folate deficiency
—pregnancy (although we question the validity of this finding, because it is possible that B$_{12}$ deficiency is under-recognized in pregnancy)
—multiple myeloma
—excessive vitamin C intake
—transcobalamin I deficiency

Urinary MMA/Creatinine Ratio Test

1. Elevated in vitamin B$_{12}$ deficiency
2. Elevated in some inborn errors of B$_{12}$ metabolism
3. Highly sensitive
4. Highly specific
    (No known false positive or false negative results)

5. Adjusts for poor renal function
6. Adjusts for hypovolemia/dehydration
7. Non-invasive
8. No fasting required (spot urine)
9. Cost-effective

Serum MMA

1. Elevated in vitamin B_{12} deficiency
2. Elevated in certain inborn errors of B_{12} metabolism
3. Falsely high in renal insufficiency
4. Falsely high in intravascular volume depletion
5. Twelve-hour fasting required
6. Invasive
7. Less sensitive and specific than urinary MMA

Plasma Homocysteine

1. Elevated in vitamin B_{12} deficiency
2. Elevated in folate deficiency
3. Elevated in vitamin B_6 deficiency
4. Elevated in renal insufficiency
5. Elevated in intravascular volume depletion
6. Elevated in chronic diseases (hypothyroidism, systemic lupus erythematosus, severe psoriasis, some cancers, renal failure)
7. Elevated with the use of specific medications (Dilantin, Tegretol, nitrous oxide, methotrexate, lipid-lowering drugs [colestipol and niacin in combination with thiazide diuretics], estrogen-containing oral contraceptives).
8. Elevated in inherited errors of methionine metabolism:

—cystathionine ß-synthase deficiency
—methionine synthase deficiency
—methylenetetrahydrofolate reductase deficiency

9. Elevated in certain inborn errors of B_{12} metabolism
10. Twelve-hour fasting required
11. Invasive

The History of the Urinary MMA

By 1967, researchers knew that elevated urinary MMA revealed B$_{12}$ deficiency. However, because testing for urinary MMA was laborious and time-consuming at that time, urinary MMA was not adopted as a clinical procedure.

What clinicians needed was a sensitive and rapid test measuring MMA in the urine—a test that was developed in 1982 by researcher Eric J. Norman, Ph.D., in collaboration with the late Dr. M. Drue Denton and coworkers at the Hematology Division of the University of Cincinnati College of Medicine. Dr. Norman's laboratory team developed an assay for urinary MMA using a gas chromatography/mass spectrometric (GC/MS) method that was fast, sensitive, and reproducible. In tests involving nearly 2,000 subjects with megaloblastic anemia, other anemias, elevated red cell mean corpuscular volume, or unexplained neurologic disorders, the researchers found that the urinary MMA test was a better indicator of B$_{12}$ deficiency than the serum B$_{12}$, the Schilling test, and other basic hematologic tests. They also found that many patients without anemia had already suffered permanent neurologic disability due to a delay in diagnosis—stemming, in a number of cases, from the lack of accurate tests.

By 1985, the urinary MMA/creatinine ratio test was perfected, and Dr. Norman and his wife Claudia opened their own laboratory (Norman Clinical Laboratory) to provide low-cost test kits for B$_{12}$ screening. Around this time a separate research group, studying Dr. Norman's data and research, analyzed stored blood samples from patients with pernicious anemia and other types of B$_{12}$ deficiency and also concluded that MMA testing was superior to serum B$_{12}$ tests. The results of this study were published in the *New England Journal of Medicine* in 1988.[12]

Despite this early confirmation of the value of the urinary MMA, the medical community has made only minimal use of this important screening tool. Although the test is far more accurate than other tests, including the serum MMA (see chart earlier in this chapter), and is inexpensive as well, very few physicians order urinary MMAs for patients suspected of having B$_{12}$ deficiency. It is our hope that as clinicians and researchers become more knowledgeable about the scope and consequences of B$_{12}$ deficiency, they also will become more aware of the need to include the highly sensitive and accurate urinary MMA as part of their screening protocol.

proper diagnostic codes are used (see Appendix S). Thus, there is no financial disincentive for ordering them. If either the MMA or Hcy levels are elevated, or if the cobalamin level itself is low, proper follow-up and treatment must be initiated.

Recommended protocol for treating B_{12} deficiency

There are three forms of supplemental vitamin B_{12}: cyanocobalamin, hydroxocobalamin, and methylcobalamin. (We will review the advantages and disadvantages of the different forms shortly.) Different recommendations exist for initial and maintenance vitamin B_{12} therapy. Of these, one of the most common recommendations is the following:

- Initial intramuscular injections of vitamin B_{12}, 1,000 mcg daily or every other day for five to seven days, followed by
- Additional intramuscular injections of 1,000 mcg weekly for four weeks, followed by
- Maintenance intramuscular injections of 1,000 mcg every month. This maintenance therapy must be lifelong.

Using the regimen outlined above, hematologic improvements typically commence within five to seven days, and the deficiency should resolve after three to four weeks of therapy. If B_{12} deficiency is long-standing, and neurological manifestations are present, it can take six months or longer before signs of improvement appear. In cases where neurologic signs and symptoms have been present for a year or longer, or where impairment is severe, neurologic damage may be permanent. (This often happens when patients' laboratory results do not show macrocytic anemia, or fall into the low range of "normal" B_{12}, leading their physicians to miss the correct diagnosis for a longer period of time.) Overall, neurological symptoms are completely resolved in about half of the cases, while residual deficits remain in the other half; however, nearly all patients improve to some degree.

Treatment consists of injectable vitamin B_{12} to replace daily losses and refill storage pools. These storage pools normally contain 2 to 5 mg of vitamin B_{12}. It is thought that doses greater than 100 mcg saturate transcobalamin, and the rest is lost in the urine. Toxicity of B_{12} injections is nil, except for extremely rare allergic reactions; the only exception, discussed later in this chapter, involves patients with Leber's hereditary optic neuropathy, a very uncommon disease, in which the use of cyano-cobalamin is contraindicated.

G. Richard Lee, M.D., notes in *Wintrobe's Clinical Hematology* that a single injection, even of massive amounts of B$_{12}$, is not sufficient to replenish body stores. This is because the body's ability to retain the injected B$_{12}$ is limited. Thus, he notes, "If greater than 1 mg of B$_{12}$ is to be stored, several injections separated by at least twenty-four hours need to be administered, rather than a single dose." Lee also notes that some people are "short responders," whose serum B$_{12}$ concentrations may drop to dangerously low levels within two weeks of an injection.

During initial treatment, serum potassium concentration may fall significantly within the first forty-eight hours after an injection, and then gradually rise to normal levels over the next few weeks. Patients with borderline or low potassium levels should receive potassium supplements before therapy is initiated, to protect against arrhythmias. Temporary drops in plasma iron levels may also occur, and a transient increase in paresthesias is sometimes experienced. Hypokalemia and thrombocytosis could occur upon conversion of severe megaloblastic to normal erythropoiesis with B12 therapy. Therefore, serum potassium levels and the platelet count should be monitored during therapy.

The oral versus injected issue

There are studies noting that high-dose oral cyanocobalamin (1,000-2,000 mcg daily) is equivalent to cyanocobalamin injections. A recent U.S. study, for example, demonstrated that high-dose oral B$_{12}$ (2,000 mcg) was as effective in producing hematologic and neurologic responses as a standard injectable regimen in patients with B$_{12}$ deficiency. This study strongly supports the view that oral B$_{12}$ at doses of 2,000 mcg can replace injection therapy in *some* situations. Although this was a very small study with only thirty-three patients, it did use MMA and Hcy markers, demonstrating a reduction in these two metabolites.[13]

This study is consistent with findings from the 1950s and 1960s, which showed that 1 percent of the oral B$_{12}$ dose consumed is absorbed via an alternate pathway, irrelevant of intrinsic factor or a functioning ileum. It also is consistent with clinical practice in Sweden, where oral B$_{12}$ maintenance therapy has been used for more than twenty-five years.

However, we believe that additional research is needed to confirm the efficacy and safety of oral B_{12} for patients whose deficiencies stem from a variety of etiologies. Studies also need to be conducted comparing oral methylcobalamin to oral cyanocobalamin, and comparing injectable hydroxocobalamin and methylcobalamin to oral and injectable cyanocobalamin (see next section). It is also important to note that oral and sublingual B_{12} formulations are not regulated by the Food and Drug Administration.

Emmanuel Andres, M.D., noted recently in the *Annals of Pharmacotherapy*, "As Lane and Rojas-Fernandez demonstrated, to date only case reports or small studies have focused on oral vitamin B_{12} therapy for the treatment of cobalamin deficiencies. Thus, the ideal doses of oral cobalamin and treatment duration remain to be determined.... In several studies, cobalamin deficiency is not well established, be it low serum vitamin B_{12} concentrations or true cobalamin deficiency with biological or clinical features; nor is the etiology known, be it nutritional deficiency, pernicious anemia, or food-cobalamin malabsorption. To our knowledge, these limitations involve major difficulties with interpretation of the data."[14] Lane and Rojas-Fernandez concluded in their summary, "There are inadequate data at the present time to support the use of oral cyanocobalamin replacement in patients with severe neurologic involvement."[15] We ourselves have seen cases in which injected B_{12} resulted in far greater benefits than oral supplementation.

It is true that B_{12} deficiency caused by food-cobalamin malabsorption can be treated with high-dose oral B_{12} (1,000 mcg daily). Unfortunately, doctors may fail to accurately determine which patients fall into this category, and the assumption that all elderly patients have B_{12} deficiency caused by food malabsorption will endanger those with other conditions. In addition, physicians prescribing oral B_{12} must be aware that while the bottle label on B_{50} complex tells the physician and the patient that it contains 833 percent of the percent daily value, it contains only 50 mcg of B_{12}. Centrum Silver multivitamins contain only 25 mcg of B_{12}, and typical multivitamins contain only 6 mcg. These amounts are grossly inadequate for patients who have malabsorption problems and need to ingest 1,000 mcg of oral B_{12} daily.

Moreover, even in cases of malabsorption, relying on oral supplementation may delay or eliminate the use of injections for patients who would otherwise benefit from having their stores rapidly replenished. Further, in cases involving patients who are non-compliant or suffer from memory problems or mental illness, injections administered in the office or by a family member are far more reliable than oral supplements which patients may forget to take. Also, some patients object to taking an increased number of oral medications, while others have problems swallowing tablets, or have sensitive stomachs and can easily be nauseated by oral supplements. (High-dose sublingual B$_{12}$ may be an option for these patients.)

With the development of virtually painless microfine needles, the only significant drawback to injected B$_{12}$—injection pain—has been greatly reduced. Moreover, patients can easily learn to inject themselves, making injected B$_{12}$ much less expensive than oral supplements.

The argument for injections is simple: Given that injectable B$_{12}$ is safe, effective, inexpensive, and virtually painless (and also eliminates the issue of compliance if shots are administered at the physician's office), why take a chance on oral formulations that may not be as effective? In cases of temporary B$_{12}$ deficiency due solely to poor diet, however, oral supplementation is, of course, effective, once normal B$_{12}$ levels have been reestablished and any other reasons for the deficiency have been carefully ruled out.

Which form of cobalamin is best?

Current evidence indicates that hydroxocobalamin is superior to cyanocobalamin, and methylcobalamin may be superior to hydroxocobalamin for neurologic disease. Lee notes in *Wintrobe's Clinical Hematology*, "The initial retention of hydroxocobalamin is better than that of cyanocobalamin; twenty-eight days after injection, retention still is nearly three times greater. In addition, hydroxocobalamin is more available to cells and is processed more efficiently by them."

Methylcobalamin (available at compound pharmacies, with or without preservatives) is not yet widely used in the United States, but Japanese studies indicate that it is even more effective in treating neurological sequelae of B$_{12}$ deficiency. Its greater efficacy presumably stems at least in part from the fact that, like hydroxocobalamin, it does not need to be decyanated—and, in addition, unlike either hydroxocobalamin or cyanocobalamin, it does not need to be reduced to the (+1) state (the only form that can cross the blood-brain barrier). Thus, it bypasses several potentially problematic stages in B$_{12}$ metabolism. Furthermore, methylcobalamin provides the body with methyl groups essential for various biological oxidation-reduction reactions. Studies show that a small oral dose of methylcobalamin results in a greater accumulation of cobalamin in the liver than an oral dose of cyanocobalamin, and that methylcobalamin is retained approximately three times longer in tissues than cyanocobalamin.

Some concerns have been raised about using a cyanide-based vitamin B_{12} derivative. Patients with Leber's hereditary optic neuropathy (LHON) should *never* receive cyanocobalamin; LHON is associated with an inability to properly clear cyanide from the body, and there is evidence that the optic atrophy associated with LHON can be exacerbated by the administration of cyanocobalamin. (Hydroxocobalamin and methylcobalamin can, of course, be used to treat LHON patients, as they do not contain the cyano-group [cyanide]. In fact, there is evidence that some cases of optic neuropathy respond dramatically to hydroxocobalamin, which acts as a cyanide antagonist.)

People with hepatic dysfunction also can have elevated cyanide levels, and children with inborn errors of B_{12} metabolism may have a metabolic defect involving cyanide metabolism. Smokers, too, have elevated cyanide levels, and research shows that hydroxocobalamin injections can decrease smokers' blood cyanide levels by 59 percent; conversely, administration of cyanocobalamin could potentially raise the cyanide levels of smokers.[16]

Given the greater safety of hydroxocobalamin and methylcobalamin, as well as their greater effectiveness, we agree with physician Steve Roach, who says, "I would not expect any adverse effects in most patients with either preparation [cyanocobalamin or hydroxocobalamin]. However, it seems wise to avoid a potentially harmful form of a drug when the more physiologic variety is available and is excreted at a more desirable rate."[17] In light of the current evidence, we suggest hydroxocobalamin over cyanocobalamin for the treatment of typical pernicious anemia patients, as well as patients with neurologic symptoms resulting from delayed diagnosis. Recent research has found that patients with neurologic involvement may benefit even more from high-dose methylcobalamin.[18]

No matter which form of cobalamin is used, it is crucial to make any of your patients who need long-term treatment, such as those with a history of gastric surgery, aware of the need to continue treatment for life. It is important, too, to provide them with documentation that will make it easier for them to obtain treatment in the future, if they need to switch doctors. Also, encourage the hospitals with which you are affiliated to develop protocols for effective B$_{12}$ screening. B$_{12}$ deficiency is a public health crisis, and it is crucial—particularly as the huge Baby Boomer generation ages—that we develop appropriate standards of care in order to acknowledge, address, and handle this crisis.

Cost-Effective

We find that prescribing a 30 ml vial of hydroxocobalamin 1,000 mcg/ml works well for patients self-administering their B$_{12}$. The cost is approximately $38 if a patient has no insurance, and the cost of a co-pay for patients with insurance. One bottle will last two years or less, depending on the expiration date. The bottle needs to be stored between 59 to 86 degrees Fahrenheit. Unfortunately, pharmaceutical companies do not make 10 ml vials of hydroxocobalamin, but this may change in the future. Cyanocobalamin is supplied in either 1 ml vials ($1.00 per vial of 1,000 mcg/ml) or 10 ml vials ($10.00 per 10 ml vial of 1,000 mcg/ml). (Prices are 2005.)

An obligation for all specialties

We're often told, as emergency department (ED) staff, that comprehensive testing for B$_{12}$ deficiency is inappropriate in our setting. Yet a significant percentage of our "repeaters"—the patients who come in month after month suffering from mental status changes, syncope, chest pain, anemia, weakness, dizziness, or fractures caused by falls—are likely to be suffering from a B$_{12}$ deficiency that is causing or exacerbating their health problems.

We believe that the ED is an appropriate place for B$_{12}$ testing. We have an ethical obligation to rule out B$_{12}$ deficiency in ED patients who present with high-risk signs and symptoms, and we've saved the health and lives of many patients by doing this, so we encourage ED staff to order tests when indicated—but ideally, this diagnosis should occur in the office of a primary care physician or specialist who can provide long-term follow-up.

B$_{12}$ deficiency is a problem that should be identified and treated long before it causes symptoms serious enough to require emergency care. In the great majority of cases, B$_{12}$ deficiency develops slowly, and it can easily be diagnosed months or even years before it causes painful or dangerous symptoms.

Early diagnosis and treatment can become the norm, if doctors in every specialty take responsibility for identifying patients deficient in B_{12}. The neurologist whose patient complains of dizziness or neuropathy or pain; the psychiatrist whose patient is depressed or paranoid or psychotic; the gynecologist whose patient continues to have abnormal Pap smears or infertility; the gastroenterologist caring for patients with Crohn's disease, celiac disease or other GI disorders; the cardiologist treating patients with heart attacks, congestive heart failure, and hyperhomocysteinemia; the endocrinologist who sees patients with thyroid and other autoimmune disorders, and patients with neuropathy seemingly related to diabetes; the orthopedic surgeon who treats patients with fall-related fractures; the anesthesiologist treating chronic pain and fibromyalgia patients, or administering nitrous oxide to at-risk patients; the pediatrician or pediatric neurologist treating children with mental retardation or symptoms resembling autism—all must realize that complete B_{12} testing is a crucial part of a thorough workup.

Very rarely in medicine can a severely debilitating and potentially life-threatening disorder be so easily diagnosed, and so easily and inexpensively treated. The doctor who fails to screen patients with suspicious symptoms or histories for B_{12} deficiency will indeed save a few minutes, and one to two hundred dollars worth of tests in the short run, but he or she almost certainly will also be condemning some of these patients to severe debility—and condemning the health-care system to the financial burden of caring for them. Conversely, the wise doctor who remembers to include B_{12} deficiency in a differential diagnosis whenever symptoms warrant will save both health-care dollars and patients' lives.

Moreover, doctors who look diligently for B_{12} deficiency often save the lives of their own loved ones. One of us (J. S.), initially skeptical about routinely testing for B_{12} deficiency, changed his mind when he discovered that it affected not just many of his patients but four members of his own family as well. Luckily, he diagnosed them in time to protect their health. Since then, we've convinced a number of colleagues to have relatives tested, and many have come back to us saying, "You were right, the tests showed B_{12} deficiency—thank you!"

A thoracic surgeon, writing in the *Journal of the American Medical Association*, wasn't as lucky. His wife suffered severe and probably irreversible neurological symptoms, because a number of specialists missed her B$_{12}$ deficiency. "Her experiences with competent physicians at a major medical center convinced me that vitamin B$_{12}$ deficiency is not a benign condition, and it is not diagnosed easily by general physicians," he wrote.[19] But it is easy to diagnose. Unfortunately, it's also easily overlooked by doctors who are uninformed about B$_{12}$ deficiency and its deadly consequences. These physicians are failing not only their patients, but even their own families, friends, and colleagues.

In contrast, physicians willing to learn about this widespread problem and share their knowledge with others are our best hope for confronting the growing problem of B$_{12}$ deficiency. One of these doctors is David Spence, M.D., who wrote in *The Lancet*[20] about his own misdiagnosis when he developed B$_{12}$ deficiency. His neurologist, noting that his B$_{12}$ level was "normal" (reference range 150-800 pmol/L. Spence's level 200 pmol/L, which, in our opinion, is actually too low.), concluded that Spence's neuropathy and other marked neurological abnormalities stemmed from an old neck injury. Spence himself concluded that his troubling, unexplained neuropathy and myelopathy probably were due to an occult malignancy, and he spent six months worrying about this possibility.

By luck, however, Spence's personal interest and study regarding homocysteine and vascular disease led him to begin taking high-dose B vitamins, including 500 mcg of B$_{12}$ daily, around this time. His lab results revealed that he had a high homocysteine level (a natural consequence of his undiagnosed B$_{12}$ deficiency), and he was aware of the vitamin's effects in lowering homocysteine. When his neuropathy began improving, and when a follow-up test showed that his serum B$_{12}$ level was still in the low normal range—at a time when it should have been very high, due to the fairly high dose of oral B$_{12}$ he was taking—the correct diagnosis dawned on him: "It was clear that I was malabsorbing vitamin B$_{12}$." As it turned out, his problem involved a defect of transcobalamin II, a protein needed to transport B$_{12}$ once it crosses the ileal mucosa.

Spence now makes every effort to inform physicians about the widespread phenomenon of B$_{12}$ deficiency and its consequences. "I am working on reducing the prevalence of this knowledge gap," he says, citing a quotation from William Osler: "It is the obligation and the joy of the physician to be a perpetual student."

Osler's quote is indeed apt, because the current epidemic of B$_{12}$ deficiency presents physicians with both a tremendous obligation—the obligation to combat this epidemic—and a tremendous opportunity to conduct exciting research in an area of medicine that is in desperate need of more study. Indeed, it is remarkable, given the destruction that B_{12} deficiency wreaks on so many body systems—hematologic, neurologic, cardiovascular, reproductive, gastrointestinal, musculoskeletal—that so many questions about the disorder remain unanswered. Medical professionals interested in clinical or laboratory research would be well advised to aid in bridging this knowledge gap, by making research on B_{12} deficiency a priority. Among the issues that researchers need to address are the following:

- What percent of fractures in elderly patients who fall are caused by undiagnosed B_{12} deficiency?
- What percentage of diabetics have peripheral neuropathy caused in part by B_{12} deficiency?
- What percentage of patients who experience transient ischemic attacks, strokes, chest pain, or congestive heart failure have underlying B_{12} deficiency? (See Chapter 5.)
- What percentage of patients with dementia or Alzheimer's are deficient in B_{12}, causing dementia-like symptoms? (See Chapter 2.)
- What percentage of patients institutionalized or admitted to outpatient psychiatric facilities have low B_{12}? (See Chapter 4.)
- Postoperative patients often suffer complications, ranging from weakness, paresthesias, or paralysis to depression and memory loss. How often are these symptoms due to untreated B_{12} deficiency which was exacerbated by exposure to nitrous oxide during surgery and/or increased metabolic demands and tissue repair after surgery? (See Chapter 8.)
- What is the rate of B_{12} deficiency among infertile men and women? What percentage of women with abnormal Pap smears are B_{12}-deficient? (See Chapter 9 for more on both.)
- What percent of AIDS patients with neuropathy or dementia actually have neurological symptoms due to untreated B_{12} deficiency, a common condition in AIDS patients? (See Chapter 7.)
- How many motor vehicle accidents (particularly among the elderly) involve B_{12} deficiency, which often causes confusion, dizziness, slowed reflexes, and neuropathy that can leave

sufferers unable to control a vehicle's gas and brake pedals, or cause poor judgment behind the wheel? (See Chapter 2.)

- How many dialysis patients have B$_{12}$ deficiency? Does giving hydroxocobalamin or methylcobalamin (IM or IV) decrease these patients' elevated MMA and Hcy levels and aid in treating uremic neuropathy? (Recent studies indicate the answer is "yes."[21]) (See Chapter 5.)

- How many children diagnosed with "autism" actually have an undiagnosed inborn error of B$_{12}$ metabolism, a defect in the transport of B$_{12}$, or an acquired B$_{12}$ deficiency due to environmental factors? (See Chapter 12.)

We strongly encourage teaching hospitals and other medical facilities to put research into these issues at the very top of their "to do" lists. Answers to these critical questions will aid us in bringing the hidden epidemic of B$_{12}$ deficiency out into the open, identifying all of its victims, and offering them the help they so desperately need.

A quiz for physicians: Did you know these facts about vitamin B$_{12}$ deficiency?

1. Vitamin B$_{12}$ deficiency and/or pernicious anemia may be present without anemia or macrocytosis.

2. Vitamin B$_{12}$ deficiency and/or pernicious anemia may be present in patients with a normal CBC or a microcytic anemia.

3. Patients with B$_{12}$ deficiency have been misdiagnosed as having anemia of chronic disease and internal bleeding. After extensive testing proves no bleeding has occurred, patients are given the diagnosis of "unexplained anemia."

4. In the past, by the time anemia was symptomatic, more than 80 percent of patients had neurologic manifestations, and in 50 percent this led to some permanent incapacity.

5. Patients have acquired permanent neurological damage because of delayed diagnosis or misdiagnosis.

6. Patients with B$_{12}$ deficiency have been confined to wheelchairs or bedridden because of chronic misdiagnosis.

7. Permanent spastic gait or paralysis can result from misdiagnosed B$_{12}$ deficiency.

8. Peripheral neuropathy occurs in about 25 percent of untreated patients.

9. Subtle changes in mental status are present in as many as two-thirds of patients before treatment is started.

10. Urinary MMA testing is superior to basic serum B_{12} tests and is needed to assist in diagnosis.

11. Patients with vitamin B_{12} deficiency have been misdiagnosed with diabetic neuropathy.

12. Patients with B_{12} deficiency/pernicious anemia have been misdiagnosed with multiple sclerosis.

13. Patients with B_{12} deficiency have been misdiagnosed with dementia and wrongfully placed in nursing homes.

14. Patients with B_{12} deficiency have been misdiagnosed with psychiatric disorders.

15. Vitamin B_{12} deficiency is found in all ages, from infants to geriatrics, and in all ethnic groups.

16. Research indicates that B_{12} deficiency affects one of every seven seniors. Some studies indicate that the number is even higher, with up to 25 percent of the elderly suffering from undiagnosed B_{12} deficiency.

17. Emergency medicine physicians encounter undiagnosed or misdiagnosed B_{12}-deficient patients every day in their current practice.

18. Vitamin B_{12} deficiency causes hyperhomocysteinemia, which leads to an increased risk of strokes, MIs, DVTs, and PEs.

19. B_{12} deficiency causes dizziness, imbalance, and orthostatic hypotension.

20. Many elderly patients who have fallen and sustained fractures have been found to be B_{12}-deficient.

21. Patients administered nitrous oxide during surgery or dental procedures can have poor outcomes and even death if they have undiagnosed B_{12} deficiency preoperatively.

22. Patients two to six weeks post-op who complain of paresthesias, TIA symptoms, frequent falls, and/or mental status changes could have nitrous oxide-induced myelopathy due to undiagnosed B_{12} deficiency.

23. Vitamin B_{12} deficiency is easy to diagnose and inexpensive to treat, and testing is reimbursable.

24. Costly malpractice suits have resulted from failure to diagnose B_{12} deficiency.

25. Early diagnosis of B$_{12}$ deficiency would help the health care budget deficit by dramatically reducing ED, hospital, rehabilitation, home care, and nursing home usage.

26. Billions of dollars could be saved with early diagnosis.

27. There is a critical window of opportunity for treating B$_{12}$ deficiency before irreversible neurological damage results.

Notes

1. Dharmarajan, T. S., and Norkus, E. P. Approaches to vitamin B$_{12}$ deficiency: Early treatment may prevent devastating complications. *Postgraduate Medicine* 2001;110(1); 99–105.

2. Ibid.

3. Antony, A. C. Megaloblastic anemias. In R. Hoffman et al. (3rd Ed.), *Hematology: Basic Principles and Practice* (pp. 457–467). 2000, Philadelphia: Churchill, Livingstone; and Savage, D. G., Lindenbaum, J., Stabler, S. P., and Allen, R. H. Sensitivity of serum methylmalonic acid and total homocysteine determinations for diagnosing cobalamin and folate deficiencies. *American Journal of Medicine* 1994, 96:239–246; and Norman, E. J., and Morrison, J. A. Screening elderly populations for cobalamin (vitamin B$_{12}$) deficiency using the urinary methylmalonic acid assay by gas chromatography mass spectrometry. *American Journal of Medicine* 1993, 94:589–594; and Stabler, S. P., Lindenbaum, J., and Allen, R. H. The use of homocysteine and other metabolites in the specific diagnosis of vitamin B$_{12}$ deficiency. *Journal of Nutrition* 1996, 126:1266S–1272S.

4. Dharmarajan, T. S., Norkus, E. P. Approaches to vitamin B$_{12}$ deficiency: Early treatment may prevent devastating complications. Postgraduate Medicine 2001;110(1); 99–105; and Snow, C. F. Laboratory diagnosis of vitamin B$_{12}$ and folate deficiency. *Archives of Internal Medicine* 1999;159:1289–98.

5. Shahar, A., Feiglin, L., Shahar, D. R., Levy, S., and Seligsohn, U. High prevalence and impact of subnormal serum vitamin B$_{12}$ levels in Israeli elders admitted to a geriatric hospital. *Journal of Nutrition, Health and Aging* 2001, 5(2):124–7.

6. Crane, M. G., Register, U. D., Lukens, R. H., and Gregory, R. Cobalamin (CBL) studies on two total vegetarian (vegan) families. *Vegetarian Nutrition: An International Journal* 1998, 2(3):87–92.

7. Bissoli, L., Di Francesco, V., Ballarin, A., Mandragona, R., Trespidi, R., Brocco, G., Caruso, B., Bosello, O., and Zamboni. Effect of vegetarian diet on homocysteine levels. *Annals of Nutrition and Metabolism* 2002, 46(2):73–9.

8. "B$_{12}$ deficiency may be more widespread than thought," USDA Agricultural Research Service, August 2, 2000.

9. Lee, G. R. Pernicious anemia and other causes of vitamin B$_{12}$ (cobalamin)

deficiency. In G. R. Lee (10th Ed.), *Wintrobe's Clinical Hematology*, (pp. 941–958). 1999, Baltimore: Williams & Wilkins.

10. Kalikiri, P. C., and Sachan, R. S. G. S. Nitrous oxide induced elevation of plasma homocysteine and methylmalonic acid levels and their implications. *The International Journal of Anesthesiology* 2004, 8(2).

11. Ostreicher, D. S. Vitamin B_{12} supplements as protection against nitrous oxide inhalation: *New York State Dental Journal* 1994, 60(3):47–9; and Quarnstrom, F. Nitrous oxide analgesia. What is a safe level of exposure for the dental staff? *Dentistry Today* 2002, 21(4):104–9.

12. Lindenbaum, J., et al. Neuropsychiatric disorders caused by cobalamin deficiency in the absence of anemia or macrocytosis. *New England Journal of Medicine* 1988, 318:1720–8.

13. Kuzminski, A. M., et al. Effective treatment of cobalamin deficiency with oral cobalamin. *Blood* 1998, 92(4):1191–8.

14. Andrès, E. Comment: Treatment of vitamin B_{12} deficiency anemia: Oral versus parenteral therapy. *Annals of Pharmacotherapy* 2002, 36:1268–72.

15. Lane, L. A., and Rojas-Fernandez, C. Treatment of vitamin B_{12}-deficiency anemia: oral versus parenteral therapy. *Annals of Pharmacotherapy* 2002, 36:1268–71.

16. Forsyth, J. C., et al. Hydroxocobalamin as a cyanide antidote: Safety, efficacy and pharmacokinetics in heavily smoking normal volunteers. *Journal of Toxicology and Clinical Toxicology* 1993, 31(2):277–94.

17. Roach, E. S., and McLean, W. T. Neurologic disorders of vitamin B_{12} deficiency. *American Family Physician* 1982, 25(1):111–5.

18. Kira, J., Tobimatsu, S., and Goto, I. Vitamin B_{12} metabolism and massive-dose methyl vitamin B_{12} therapy in Japanese patients with multiple sclerosis. *Internal Medicine* 1994, 33(2):82–6.

19. Brantigan, C. O. Folate supplementation and the risk of masking vitamin B_{12} deficiency. *Journal of the American Medical Association* 1997, 277(11):884–5.

20. Spence, D. Uses of error: Knowledge gaps. *The Lancet* 2001, 358(9297):1934.

21. Kuwabara, S. et al. Intravenous methylcobalamin treatment for uremic and diabetic neuropathy in chronic hemodialysis patients. *Internal Medicine* 1999, 38(6):472–5; and Koyama, K., Usami, T., Takeuchi, O., Morozumi, K., and Kimura, G. Efficacy of methylcobalamin on lowering total homocysteine plasma concentrations in haemodialysis patients receiving high-dose folic acid supplementation. *Nephrology, Dialysis, Transplantation* 2002, 17(5):916–922; and Rostand, S. G. Vitamin B_{12} levels and nerve conduction velocities in patients undergoing maintenance hemodialysis. *American Journal of Clinical Nutrition* 1976, 29(7): 691–7.

12

Speculation: The Possible Role of Vitamin B_{12} in Autism

Vitamin B_{12} is vital for proper brain function, and deficiencies often cause mental symptoms. In particular, classic B_{12} deficiency in infants and children frequently causes symptoms similar to those seen in autism, including loss of speech and social skills. It is not uncommon, moreover, for children with identified inborn errors of B_{12} metabolism to be diagnosed as autistic before the true cause of their disorder is uncovered (see Chapter 6).

It is our belief that a significant percentage of children with autistic-like symptoms have problems which stem from unidentified disorders of B_{12} metabolism, preventing their bodies from properly using B_{12}. This hypothesis, while speculative and yet to be proven, is supported by both our personal experience and clinical reports from other physicians. Also, we cannot ignore growing evidence that some children diagnosed as autistic have true B_{12} deficiency, as proven by elevated MMAs and a positive response to B_{12} treatment (by injection).

One physician who specializes in treating autism, James Neubrander, M.D., recently reported that he is having tremendous success in treating autism, pervasive developmental disorder (PDD), and Asperger's syndrome with methylcobalamin injections. To document his success, Dr. Neubrander conducted a study using injectable methylcobalamin, involving eighty-five children diagnosed with autism spectrum disorders. Of the eighty-five children, sixty-seven had urinary MMAs performed, and forty-nine homocysteine levels were performed.

Thirteen of the sixty-seven children who received MMA testing, or

19 percent, had elevated MMAs, indicating true vitamin B_{12} deficiency. Five of the forty-nine children who received homocysteine testing, or 10 percent, had elevated homocysteine, indicating B_{12}, B_6, or folic acid deficiency or possibly an inborn error of metabolism. These abnormal results could stem from nutritional deficiencies as a result of inadequate intake, from diseases of the gastrointestinal tract, from defects in B_{12} transport, or from inborn errors of B_{12} metabolism. This study clearly indicates that some children are being misdiagnosed as autistic, when there is demonstrable evidence that they have a functional B_{12} deficiency.

What is even more interesting is that of all of the children in the study, 90 percent responded to injectable methylcobalamin, with responses ranging from mild to dramatic. Therefore, Neubrander concluded that "the current 'gold standard' lab tests documenting B_{12} deficiency, as we presently define it, have no predicative value as to which children may or may not respond to methylcobalamin therapy."[1]* (Despite Dr. Neubrander's findings, we strongly believe that all autistic children need to be tested before beginning methylcobalamin treatment to ascertain which of them have true B_{12} problems. Documentation will assist future research and aid in the development of protocols.)

Dr. Neubrander reported in June 2004 (personal communication) that he has now treated approximately 500 children and adolescents with subcutaneous methylcobalamin injections, and that nine out of ten exhibited significant improvement in symptoms. The primary symptoms parents reported as improved were language and communication, 71 percent; awareness, 65 percent; cognition and higher levels of reasoning, 52 percent; engagement, 43 percent; eye contact, 37 percent; better behavior, 35 percent; ability to focus, 35 percent; greater understanding, 35

---

* One explanation as to why some children with normal MMAs still respond to methylcobalamin injections is that they may have the inborn error of B_{12} metabolism type Cbl-E or Cbl-G. These two inborn errors of B_{12} metabolism cause elevated homocysteine but not elevated MMA, and both are responsive to vitamin B_{12} therapy. Some autistic children who are not responsive to methylcobalamin may have other inborn errors, or may have homocystinuria caused by cystathionine ß-synthase deficiency or methylene tetrahydrofolate reductase deficiency. In both of these conditions, the MMA is normal and Hcy is elevated; neither is responsive to B_{12} therapy. If adenosyl-B_{12} coenzyme is deficient or absent, MMA cannot be converted into succinic acid. Therefore, MMA will rise and leach out into the urine and blood, giving rise to methylmalonic aciduria.

percent; vocalization, 35 percent; and "trying new things," 33 percent. (These are the same areas in which "Billy" improved after receiving hydroxocobalamin injections—see Chapter 6.)

Arnold Brenner, M.D., has reported similar beneficial effects in many autistic patients. Improvements seen in his patients include better speech, an increased interest in reading, a decrease in hyperkinesis, and reductions in anger, hostility, and rage reactions. It is of interest that while two of Dr. Brenner's patients (as well as their mothers) were found to exhibit overt B$_{12}$ deficiency, the remainder presented with normal or even elevated levels of B$_{12}$, and none exhibited elevations in plasma homocysteine. (Unfortunately, MMAs were not performed.)[2]**

It is interesting to note that signs and symptoms of B$_{12}$ deficiency generally seen in adults can also be seen in autistic patients. For example, undiagnosed B$_{12}$ deficiency in a seventy-eight-year-old can result in behavior that includes dementia, babbling, psychosis, rocking, poor attention, and the appearance of "being in a separate world." The infant or toddler with an undiagnosed B$_{12}$ defect can also exhibit dementia, babble, have a poor attention span, appear unresponsive to the outside world, rock, or appear psychotic. The key difference between these two groups lies in their age and, thus, their stage of brain development. The adult has already acquired language, is wired for speech, and has a mature brain. The infant or toddler, in contrast, has not acquired or mastered speech or language, nor passed through all of the normal developmental stages. Therefore, the infant's or child's vocabulary and behavioral repertoire are more primitive, and symptoms will be expressed in a different way.

In short, in our opinion, senior citizens with dementia could just as accurately be labeled as "autistic," and we could just as accurately label children with autism as "demented" or "senile." In all cases of adult dementia, B$_{12}$ deficiency must be ruled out. However, we do not do this

---

** Very little formal research has been done to date on the autism/B$_{12}$ connection. The only article found on MEDLINE regarding the relationship between B$_{12}$ and autism was from 1981, entitled "Folic Acid and B$_{12}$ in Autism and Neuropsychiatric Disturbances of Childhood," in the American Academy of Childhood Psychiatry. The authors, T. L. Lowe, et al., concluded that there was no evidence of low serum B$_{12}$ or folate levels or low CSF folate in children with autism, nor did autistic children's values differ from the normal population. This study is severely flawed and outdated, because neither MMAs nor Hcys were performed.

with autistic children because the medical community has not yet made the connection between the behaviors labeled as dementia and the behaviors labeled as autism.

Of course, not all children diagnosed with autism spectrum disorder have a B$_{12}$ defect, but we believe that a significant percentage do. Given the response of autistic patients to B$_{12}$ treatment and the documentation of elevated MMA and Hcy, as reported by Dr. Neubrander, it appears the number may be around 25 percent, and perhaps even higher.

What could explain the response of many autistic children to injections of methylcobalamin? Cobalamin is the general term for compounds containing the dimethylbenzimidazolylcobamide nucleus of vitamin B$_{12}$. The most common form of prescribed B$_{12}$ is *cyanocobalamin*. The amount of cyanide in cyanocobalamin is thought to be toxicologically insignificant, but humans must clear and detoxify the cyanide molecule. After this first step, humans must reduce B$_{12}$ to its usable (+1) oxidation state (the only form that can cross the blood-brain barrier) and then enzymatically change B$_{12}$ into one of two metabolically active coenzyme forms: *adenosylcobalamin* and *methylcobalamin. If any of these steps do not take place, the brain and nervous system are deprived of vital B$_{12}$.* Serum B$_{12}$ tests can come back normal—for the B$_{12}$ is locked in the serum, and reported out as B$_{12}$ analogues—but the B$_{12}$ cannot be broken down into usable forms to be transferred to essential brain and nervous tissue.

In some cases, the body cannot successfully create the active forms of vitamin B$_{12}$ from cyanocobalamin. This problem can stem from inborn errors of metabolism, pathological changes in tissues, and/or transport defects. It is logical to assume that in such cases, the inability of B$_{12}$ to cross the blood-brain barrier could give rise to altered brain function that could in time cause autistic symptomatology (particularly since such symptomatology is strikingly similar to that seen in documented cases of pediatric and adult B$_{12}$ deficiency).

Such a deficiency would not necessarily be detected by routine evaluations. Serum B$_{12}$ tests can yield normal results in people with low levels of active B$_{12}$, not only because our current cut-off points are too low and serum B$_{12}$ tests can give false negatives, but also because serum B$_{12}$ tests do not distinguish between cyanocobalamin and the active forms adenosylcobalamin and methylcobalamin.

One piece of evidence strongly implicating defects of B$_{12}$ metabolism in autism is the finding that many autistic children are found to have a glutathione deficiency. The first step in converting inactive B$_{12}$ to active methyl- or adenosylcobalamin is thought to be dependent on glutathione. It is plausible that some autistic children have a defect in converting cyanocobalamin, and thus are using up large amounts of glutathione in the conversion process. Alternately, a simple glutathione deficiency may result in a functional B$_{12}$ deficiency, because glutathione is needed to decyanate B$_{12}$.

Interestingly, there is evidence (although controversial) to indicate that a number of autistic children develop symptoms of the disorder following exposure to thimerosal, a vaccine preservative that is approximately 50 percent mercury. (Today, the use of thimerosal is generally being phased out in vaccines administered to children.) Should the association between thimerosal and autism be proven, it raises an obvious question: Why do some children who receive mercury vaccinations have an adverse reaction, when millions of other children don't? Genetic predisposition, of course, plays a part. Another key piece of evidence is that when mercury is introduced into the body, B$_{12}$ will bind to it in order to remove it. Do the children who react adversely to mercury-containing vaccines have undetected B$_{12}$ deficiency or B$_{12}$ defects, and is their B$_{12}$ deficiency worsened when exposure to mercury causes additional stores to bind to the mercury and be removed from circulation? This would be similar to the adverse response of a B$_{12}$-deficient child given nitrous oxide, which inactivates B$_{12}$.

Our theory is that immunizations with mercury tax the systems of genetically vulnerable children (those who have undiagnosed inborn errors of B$_{12}$ metabolism, B$_{12}$ transport defects, and/or B$_{12}$ deficiency), causing further depletion of already-low B$_{12}$ stores and leading to the appearance of autistic-like symptoms that are similar in many ways to the symptoms seen in B$_{12}$-deficient adults. This depletion or inactivation of B$_{12}$ is exacerbated in children who have surgeries in which nitrous oxide is administered, such as ear tube insertion, tonsillectomy, or circumcision repair. Our speculation is supported by the findings of researcher Richard Deth, Ph.D., and colleagues, who reported in 2004 that thimerosal interferes with folate-dependent methylation by inhibiting the biosynthesis of the active form of vitamin B$_{12}$ (methylcobalamin)—the form of B$_{12}$ that Dr. Neubrander and many other doctors are using with great success to treat autistic children.[3]

While the reasons many autistic children respond to methylcobalamin remain to be determined, the positive results seen in many cases—as well as the safety and inexpensiveness of B_{12} injections—make a clear case for offering methylcobalamin therapy to patients with autistic spectrum disorders. We recommend that every child with the diagnosis of autistic spectrum disorder receive testing for urinary MMA and plasma homocysteine.*** We also recommend testing before treatment to aid in determining the underlying reasons certain individuals respond to treatment, and also to determine if those with abnormal test results respond significantly better than those who have normal lab results.

Because it is impossible to predict the different variables leading towards inefficient utilization, conversion, or transport of B_{12}, injections appear to be necessary. Methylcobalamin is the chosen form, for several of the following reasons:

1. Methylcobalamin does not need to go through the decyanation process as does cyanocobalamin.
2. Methylcobalamin has an advantage over both cyanocobalamin and hydroxocobalamin, in that the body does not need to reduce the +3 and +2 forms into the +1 state.
3. Methylcobalamin also provides the body with more methyl groups for various chemical reactions (oxidation-reduction).

We must stress that B_{12} therapy is not a cure-all, which is one reason urinary MMA and Hcy must be tested. To us, it only makes sense to treat the individual rather than the group, because a treatment that benefits one child may not help another. Some inborn errors of metabolism

---

*** Researchers have proposed that there are approximately four steps required to convert cyanocobalamin to the active coenzyme forms (methylcobalamin and adenosylcobalamin). (Pezacka, E., Green, R., and Jacobsen, D. W. Glutathionylcobalamin as an intermediate in the formation of cobalamin coenzymes. *Biochem* Biophys Res Comm 1990, 2:443–50.) Methylcobalamin is found in blood plasma, cerebral spinal fluid, and in the cytosol of cells. Adenosylcobalamin predominates in cellular tissues, where it is retained in the mitochondria. If there is a defect not allowing the conversion of cyanocobalamin to methylcobalamin, B_{12} is not in its usable form, and is limited or unusable in the blood plasma, cerebral spinal fluid, and the cytosol of cells. We speculate that this breakdown of the normal B_{12} pathway involves a genetic defect of B_{12} metabolism that is responsible for some cases of autism and multiple sclerosis.

will not respond to B$_{12}$, but because B$_{12}$, B$_6$ and folic acid share common pathways, it is possible that giving megadoses of B$_{12}$ will sometimes aid in alleviating the effects of other errors. Some children may respond to B$_6$ (a commonly used autism therapy) because of these common pathways, when the actual defect involves B$_{12}$, or vice versa.**** Guessing at which essential vitamin is needed and administering the wrong one (or an inappropriate dose) during critical brain development is poor practice, when testing can potentially elucidate the underlying problem and its correct treatment.

In summary, the reasons autistic children could be B$_{12}$ deficient or have a B$_{12}$ defect include the following:

1. B$_{12}$ is not crossing the blood-brain barrier.
2. B$_{12}$ is being used up because of glutathione deficiency.
3. B$_{12}$ is being used up or inactivated because of other insults (mercury, nitrous oxide).
4. B$_{12}$ cannot be absorbed because of diseased tissues of the gastrointestinal tract.
5. B$_{12}$ is not being used properly because of enzyme defects and defects in proteins transporting B$_{12}$. These defects can be complete or partial.
6. B$_{12}$ deficiency is present because of poor diet, or a prenatal deficiency caused by a vegan mother, a mother with undiagnosed pernicious anemia, or a mother with B$_{12}$ deficiency due to other causes. This is worsened if the mother had breast-fed the child.
7. The amount of B$_{12}$ in prenatal vitamins is clearly not enough for vegans, or for women with undiagnosed B$_{12}$ deficiency.
8. In today's weight-conscious society, many pregnant women do not eat foods rich in vitamin B$_{12}$.

**** For instance, about half of all cystathionine ß-synthase-deficient patients respond to large doses of pyridoxine (vitamin B$_6$) with marked decreases in homocystinemia, homocystinuria, and hypermethioninemia. The capacity to so respond is genetically determined and usually correlates with the presence of at least a trace of residual activity of cystathionine ß-synthase. The response is thought to be mediated by a few-fold increase in such residual activity. Restoration of activity to normal is not necessary to obtain a detectable response. From such cases, we learn one basis for cofactor (vitamin) therapies.

A final note: No discussion of inborn errors of metabolism in autism would be complete without mentioning the work of researcher Bernard Rimland, Ph.D., who was the first to discover the connection between autism and another vitamin—vitamin B_6, or pyridoxine—thirty years ago. Since then, eighteen consecutive studies, conducted by researchers in six countries, have revealed that almost 50 percent of all autistic children and adults responded favorably to high doses of B_6 and magnesium, with no adverse effects reported. Eleven of these studies were double-blind, placebo-controlled experiments. It should come as no surprise that both vitamin B_6 and vitamin B_{12} deficiencies are linked to autism, and that folate deficiencies have also been implicated. As we have noted throughout this book, these three nutrients play crucial and intertwined roles in metabolic pathways essential to mental and physical health.

Questions about autism and B_{12} that need to be answered:

1. Do the children who respond with a greater reversal in signs and symptoms of autistic behavior have elevated MMA and Hcy? What percentage of children diagnosed with autism have elevated MMAs? What percentage have elevated Hcy? What percentage have both elevated MMA and Hcy?

2. Does response in symptoms depend on age? Is there a critical period of brain development during which untreated defects in B_{12} metabolism will cause permanent neurological disability or mental impairment?

3. Is there a limited window of opportunity for effectively treating autistic individuals who are found to have functional B_{12} deficiency? This may be similar to dementia caused by B_{12} deficiency, in which treatment implemented after a long period of deficiency may have little or no benefit, while treatment implemented early on can result in a complete cure.

4. Some of Dr. Neubrander's patients had normal MMA, B_{12}, and Hcy levels, but responded to injections of methylcobalamin. Could these children have transcobalamin II or R-binder deficiencies? Did the 10 percent who did not respond at all, or the others who responded mildly or moderately, possibly have cystathionine ß-synthase deficiency or methylene tetrahydrofolate reductase deficiency, for which other

therapies would be more beneficial? Do injections of methylcobalamin provide an abundance of methyl groups that may be needed to compensate for other genetic errors?

Physicians caring for developmentally disabled children should become well-versed regarding the following inborn errors of B$_{12}$ metabolism, which can cause mental retardation or autistic behavior. There is growing evidence that some children labeled as autistic have functional B$_{12}$ deficiency (proven by elevated MMA and/or Hcy). It may be possible to cure a significant number of these children, but only if they are diagnosed early.

In our opinion, all children diagnosed with autism need to be evaluated for inborn errors of B$_{12}$ metabolism. There are ten different inherited defects that are known to disrupt the pathway of B$_{12}$; three are involved in B$_{12}$ transport and seven are involved in B$_{12}$ metabolism. Some are not responsive to B$_{12}$ therapy. Thus, determining which defect is present is critical to designing an appropriate treatment plan. If testing is negative for inborn errors, a therapeutic trial of methylcobalamin injections, betaine, and other B vitamins may be used.

It is important to remember that partial defects of B$_{12}$ metabolism or transport may not present themselves until adolescence or early adulthood. This is why physicians need to rule out inborn errors of B$_{12}$ metabolism and transport defects in patients diagnosed with multiple sclerosis as well as sutism.

Inborn Errors of B_{12} Metabolism and Transport[4]

Genetic Disorders Causing Methymalonic Aciduria and /or Homocystinuria

1. Cbl-A	increase MMA	usually responsive to B_{12}	no megaloblastic anemia
2. Cbl-B	increase MMA	50 percent responsive to B_{12}	no megaloblastic anemia
3. Cbl-C	increase MMA increase Hcy	responsive to B_{12}	+ megaloblastic anemia
4. Cbl-D	increase MMA	responsive to B_{12}	unknown if megaloblastic anemia is present
5. Cbl-E (methionine synthase reductase deficiency)	increase Hcy	responsive to B_{12}	+ megaloblastic anemia
6. Cbl-F	increase MMA	responsive to B_{12}	no megaloblastic anemia
7. Cbl-G (methionine synthase deficiency)	increase Hcy	responsive to B_{12}	+ megaloblastic anemia
8. Complete mutase deficiency of enzyme methyl-malonyl CoA mutase	increase MMA	no response to B_{12}	no megaloblastic anemia
9. Partial mutase deficiency of enzyme methyl-malonyl CoA mutase	increase MMA	no response to B_{12}	no megaloblastic anemia

Homocystinuria is also caused by:

cystathionine β-synthase (CBS) deficiency	increase Hcy	not responsive to B_{12}	no megaloblastic anemia
Methylene-tetrahydrofolate reductase (MTHFR) deficiency	increase Hcy	not responsive to B12 (treatment: betaine, folate, and methionine)	no megaloblastic anemia

Cbl-A, Cbl-B, Cbl-F Methylmalonyl coenzyme A mutase deficiency (mut) disorders:

Defect in conversion of methylmalonyl coenzyme A to succinyl coenzyme A

Complete and partial mutase deficiencies: typically occur at one to four weeks of age.

Cbl-A and Cbl-B: typically occur between one and twelve months of age.

Signs and symptoms: failure to thrive, vomiting, dehydration, metabolic acidosis, muscular hypotonia, can have retarded development, hepatomegaly, hypoglycemia, coma.

—50 percent of patients present with anemia, leukopenia, thrombocytopenia

—increased MMA

Treatment: restriction of dietary amino acids that are MMA precursors (methionine, threonine, valine, and isoleucine). Complete and partial mutase deficiency of enzyme methylmalonyl CoA mutase are not responsive to B$_{12}$ therapy.

Cbl-C, Cbl-D:

Impaired synthesis of both succinyl coenzyme A and methionine, resulting in elevated MMA and Hcy.

Differentiated by genetic complementation analysis.

Cbl-C: thought to begin during the first few months of life, but a documented case was found at age four, and another at age fourteen.

Signs and symptoms: failure to thrive, poor feeding, lethargy, developmental retardation, megaloblastic anemia, some have thrombocytopenia, some have visual disturbance caused by perimacular degeneration.

—increased MMA and Hcy

Treatment: hydroxocobalamin 1,000 mcg daily, protein restriction, oral antibiotics, betaine supplements.

Cbl- E, Cbl-G:

Synthesis of homocysteine to methionine is impaired, resulting in homocystinuria and homocystinemia.

Typically patient becomes ill in the first two years of life. A delay in diagnosis may result in irreversible neurologic or developmental abnormalities.

Signs and symptoms: poor feeding, vomiting, lethargy, developmental delay, megaloblastic anemia, pancytopenia, muscular hypotonia, nystagmus, visual defects, seizures, cerebral atrophy. Documented patient became symptomatic in adulthood and was diagnosed with multiple sclerosis.

Large doses of vitamin B_{12} (hydroxocobalamin) 1,000 mcg daily need to be administered.

Abnormal vitamin B_{12} transport:

The transport protein for vitamin B_{12} is transcobalamin II (TC II). This protein must be present for the cells to accept and use vitamin B_{12}. The gene responsible for this protein is on chromosome 22. There can be an absence of TC II or abnormal TC II molecules.

TC II deficiency is a potentially deadly disease. It is typically detected within the first six to twenty weeks of life.

Signs and symptoms: weakness, diarrhea, failure to thrive, pancytopenia, megaloblastic anemia, hypogammaglobulinemia, and mucosal ulcers. Neurologic disease may present at onset or may occur later. If diagnosed late, these neurologic abnormalities may become permanent and disabling.

Serum vitamin B_{12} levels are often normal because in plasma the majority of the vitamin is bound to TC I or TC III. Some low B_{12} levels have been found in patients with other abnormalities of B_{12}-binding proteins and in the properties of TC I. Occasionally an elevated MMA or Hcy has been found.

Diagnosis is made by using chromatography or radioimmunoassay demonstrating a lack of TC II.

Treatment: Large doses of injectable hydroxocobalamin (1,000 mcg three times weekly). One child was treated orally with 2,000 mcg daily.

Some patients may have functionally abnormal TC II molecules. There appears to be a faulty protein unable to bind to B$_{12}$. Yet other patients were able to bind B$_{12}$ but could not deliver it to their cells.

Betaine is a methyl group donor that works in the normal metabolic cycle of methionine and is used to treat patients with inborn errors of methionine metabolism, because it decreases plasma homocysteine levels in the disorder homocystinuria.

Betaine is used to treat homocystinuria. It is used in the management of cystathionine β-synthase (CBS) deficiency, 5-10-methylenetetrahydrofolate reductase (MTHFR) deficiency, and certain cobalamin cofactor metabolism (*cbl*) defects. Betaine corrects elevated plasma homocysteine but does not correct the underlying basic genetic disorder. Early detection of homocystinuria in infancy and initiation of betaine therapy are essential in improving the long-term prognosis of the patient. Betaine can increase plasma concentrations of methionine and S-adenosylmethionine (SAM) in patients with homocystinuria secondary to MTHFR deficiency or *cbl* defect.

Notes

1. Presentation to the Defeat Autism Now! (DAN!) Conference, 2003.
2. Brenner, A., open letter to physicians, 1996.
3. "New research suggests link between vaccine ingredients and autism, ADHD," press release, Northeastern University, February 5, 2004.
4. Lee, G. R. Inherited and drug-induced megaloblastic anemia. In G. R. Lee (10th Ed.), *Wintrobe's Clinical Hematology*, 1999, 973-8. Baltimore: Williams & Wilkins.

13

A Call for a United Effort

In this book, we have exposed a major breakdown in America's medical system. An epidemic is raging, invisible to the public and virtually undetected by medical professionals. A safe, simple, and inexpensive cure exists, but only a minority of sufferers ever receive this treatment, or even an accurate diagnosis. As a result, hundreds of thousands of people suffer from crippling illnesses, or even lose their lives.

Clearly, action is needed to combat this epidemic. On a national scale, all of us involved in the health-care system must combat the invisible epidemic of B_{12} deficiency by standing up for the patients who count on us. This includes not only physicians, nurses, and other direct-care providers, but all others in a position to take positive action:

- Nursing home and assisted living administrators must demand accurate B_{12} testing, using the urinary MMA test, for all of their patients.
- Federal, state, and local agencies that provide medical screenings and other health-care services for the elderly need to make urinary MMA and plasma homocysteine tests part of their routine services.
- Mental health professionals and psychiatric facilities must insist on including the B_{12} screening (urinary MMA, serum B_{12}, and plasma homocysteine tests) as part of their basic workup for new patients, including those with postpartum depression or postpartum psychosis.
- Professionals treating children with developmental disabilities must understand the role that B_{12} deficiency or impaired B_{12} metabolism can play in these disorders, and they must insist on B_{12} screening for all developmentally disabled children.

- Medical insurers must allow accurate testing as a means of dramatically reducing health care expenses, rather than following the current practice of discouraging such testing—a counterproductive strategy that costs billions of dollars in the long run.
- Medical social workers must become aware of the problem of B$_{12}$ deficiency, and the role it plays in reducing patients' independence and crowding our long-term care facilities.
- Medical researchers need to study the catastrophic effects of B$_{12}$ deficiency on the elderly, including the drastically increased risk of automobile accidents due to confusion, slowed reflexes, dizziness, and hand and foot neuropathy. Should studies demonstrate a strong link between B$_{12}$ deficiency and auto accidents involving seniors, as we believe they clearly will, automobile insurance firms should insist on B$_{12}$ screening using the urinary MMA for elderly drivers.
- Government agencies responsible for promoting public health must put the problem of B$_{12}$ deficiency on their agendas, particularly with the huge Baby Boomer generation aging into the high-risk senior years.
- Consumers, too, must accept the responsibility for protecting their own health. To do this, they must insist on proper diagnosis and treatment, if they are at risk for B$_{12}$ deficiency. In addition, they must protect their loved ones—especially their children and their aging parents or grandparents—by serving as their advocates, if those in their care are in need of testing or treatment.

Together, we can stop this epidemic in its tracks. Simply by insisting on a few relatively inexpensive tests for each at-risk individual, and, for those proven to be deficient, fifteen dollars worth of B$_{12}$ injections per year. We can prevent large numbers of Americans from developing dementia or mental illness, suffering strokes or heart attacks, enduring the heartache of infertility, developing breast or cervical cancer, being crippled by developmental disabilities, or experiencing painful neuropathy or hip-fracturing falls. This is one of the most preventable, and most curable, of all medical scourges—but only if we choose to act.

Appendices

This section is intended for those who are interested in the more technical aspects of vitamin B_{12} deficiency and inborn errors of B_{12} metabolism. It may be of particular interest to medical researchers, physicians, nurses, other health-care professionals, health-care administrators, and public policy makers.

Appendix A: Causes of Vitamin B_{12} Deficiency

pernicious anemia
(autoimmunity against intrinsic
factor and/or parietal cells)

partial gastritis, gastric atrophy
(hypochlorhydria, achlorhydria)

gastrointestinal neoplasms

gastric/ileal resection (partial/total)
gastric bypass (weight loss)

malabsorption

gastric irradiation

congenital inborn metabolic errors

congenital transcobalamin II
deficiency

ileal irradiation
(bladder, cervix, uterus, prostate)

inadequate diet

veganism or vegetarianism

nitrous oxide anesthesia (surgery, dental
procedures, recreational use)

pancreatic exocrine insufficiency

Imerslund-Gräesbeck syndrome

Zollinger-Ellison syndrome

Intestinal diseases:
blind loop syndrome
celiac disease
Crohn's disease
diphyllobothrium infection
diverticulosis
gluten enteropathy
inflammatory bowel disease
small bowel overgrowth
strictures
tropical sprue

Increased demands:
chronic hemolytic anemia
hyperthyroidism
multiple myeloma
myeloproliferative disorders
neoplasms
pregnancy

Drug induced:
alcohol
antacids
biguanides:
    metformin (Glucophage)
colchicine
H2-blockers (Zantac, Tagamet, Pepcid)
proton pump inhibitors (Nexium,
    Prevacid, Prilosec, Protonix)
mycifradin sulfate (Neomycin)
phenytoin (Dilantin)
para-aminosalicylates
potassium chloride (K-Dur)
cholestyramine (Questran)

Appendix B: Systems Affected by Vitamin B$_{12}$ Deficiency

System	Pathology	Outcome

Neurologic	demyelination of CNS:
	    posterior column disease
	    lateral column disease
	    spinothalamic tract
		paresthesias, ataxia, falling, weakness, paralysis, confusion, dementia, depression, psychosis, incontinence, altered vision

Hematologic	bone marrow hypercellular megaloblastosis, hemolysis, large metamyelocytes, pancytopenia	fatigue, weakness, anemia, hepatomegaly, splenomegaly, transfusions
Immunologic	impaired DNA synthesis, leukopenia, hypersegmented neutrophils	poor wound healing, increased susceptibility to infections

Vascular	1) hyperhomocysteinemia
	
	2) enlarged heart, decreased
	    left ventricular ejection fraction
		1) occlusive vascular disorders
		    (CAD, DVT, TIA, CVA, MI)
		2) chest pain, exertional dyspnea,
		    tachycardia, palpitations, CHF

Gastrointestinal	atrophic gastritis: increased
	    goblet cells, parietal and
	    chief cell atrophy
	gastric cytology: atypical cells
	hepatomegaly
		indigestion, malabsorption, abdominal pain, weight loss, constipation, gastric stasis, increased risk of gastric cancer

Musculoskeletal	proliferation of bone marrow
	    stromal osteoprogenitors and
	    osteoblastic cells
	suppressed activity of osteoblasts
		osteoporosis and fractures in the elderly

Genitourinary	cervical dysplasia (atypical cells)
	neurogenic bladder
	    (secondary to Cbl neuropathy)
		unnecessary repeated Pap smears
		    and GYN procedures (D&C,
		    LEEP)
		unnecessary hysterectomies, recurrent cystitis
		urinary incontinence, impotence, infertility

Appendix C: Neuropsychiatric Manifestations of Vitamin B$_{12}$ Deficiency

paresthesia
weakness
gait disorder/ataxia
impaired pain perception
diminished vibratory sense
bladder/bowel incontinence
numbness
dizziness
falls
impaired fine motor coordination
diminished proprioception
muscular spasticity
abnormal reflexes
paralysis
diplopia/blurred vision

confusion/disorientation
depression
paranoia
nocturnal cramping in arms and legs
delusions
violent behavior
dementia
disturbances in taste/smell
memory loss
apathy
irritability
personality changes
hallucinations
psychosis
schizophrenia

Appendix D: Hematologic Signs
of Vitamin B$_{12}$ Deficiency

anemia	macrocytosis	anisocytosis
leukopenia	thrombocytopenia	pancytopenia
ovalocytes	neutrophil hypersegmentation	Howell-Jolly bodies

Appendix E: Signs and Symptoms
of Vitamin B$_{12}$ Deficiency

fatigue	pallor	weight loss
dizziness	congestive heart failure	loss of appetite/anorexia
lack of energy	tachycardia	sore tongue/glossitis
weakness	exertional dyspnea	diarrhea
falls	hepatomegaly	constipation
orthostatic hypotension	splenomegaly	vitiligo
gait/balance disturbances	unexplained fever	hyperpigmentation
syncope	neurologic manifestations	premature graying of hair
tinnitus	dementia/senility	psychiatric manifestations

Appendix F: Risk Factors for Developing
Vitamin B$_{12}$ Deficiency

elderly (age greater than sixty)	gastrointestinal surgery
gastrointestinal disorders/gastrointestinal cancers	hemodialysis
specific medications (Appendix A)	anesthesia/nitrous oxide administration
family history of pernicious anemia	radiation treatment
autoimmune diseases*	malnutrition

*Thyroid disorders (such as Hashimoto's thyroiditis and Graves' disease), vitiligo, Addison's disease, Type 1 diabetes, premature ovarian failure, hypoparathyroidism, hypogammaglobulinemia, agammaglobulinemia, idiopathic adrenocortical insufficiency

Appendix G: Disorders with Possible Underlying
Vitamin B$_{12}$ Deficiency

congestive heart failure	neurological disorders
iron deficiency	psychiatric disorders
anemia	demyelinating diseases (multiple sclerosis)
thrombocytopenia	peripheral neuropathies
AIDS dementia complex	hemodialysis patients
alcoholism	senility/dementia
occlusive vascular disorders	Alzheimer's disease
hyperhomocysteinemia	Parkinson's disease
autism	infertility

Appendix H: Reasons the Elderly Are at High Risk for Vitamin B12 Deficiency

atrophic gastritis
preexisting diseases
comorbid conditions
low socioeconomic status
frequent antacid use, frequently prescribed H2-blockers and proton pump inhibitors
elder discrimination
hypochlorhydria/achlorhydria
depression/isolation
alcoholism
minimizing symptoms
difficulty explaining symptoms, confusion
increased incidence of thyroid disorders
dementia
poor appetites
ill-fitting dentures/poor dentition
sore tongue/mouth
increased incidence of gastrointestinal disorders/surgeries
increased number of surgeries (nitrous oxide administration)

Appendix I: Signs and Symptoms of Vitamin B12 Deficiency Blamed on Aging or Other Factors

fatigue
neuropathy
weakness
visual disturbances
dizziness
tremor
syncope
gait disorder/ataxia
altered mental status/confusion
falling

depression
exertional dyspnea
anemia
dementia/senility
incontinence
hyperhomocysteinemia
poor wound healing
orthostatic hypotension
increased susceptibility to infections
another disorder diagnosed, therefore B12 deficiency not considered

Appendix J: Laboratory Tests to Aid in the Diagnosis of Vitamin B12 Deficiency

serum vitamin B12
parietal cell antibody
intrinsic factor antibody
peripheral blood smear
urinary methylmalonic acid (UMMA) [non-invasive]
serum methylmalonic acid (MMA)

serum gastrin
transcobalamin I, II, III
serum homocysteine (Hcy)
unsaturated B12 binding capacity
Schilling test I, II, III
gastric secretion analysis (pH)

Appendix K: Treatment Protocol for Vitamin B$_{12}$ Deficiency

Parenteral vitamin B$_{12}$ (hydroxocobalamin or cyanocobalamin)
1. 1,000mcg IM for each dose
2. Administer daily for the first week
3. Administer weekly for one month
4. Monthly injections for the remainder of patient's life

Patients may be taught to give self-injections. Variations in dosages exist because injectable B$_{12}$ is virtually non-toxic, except in very rare allergic reactions, and because of the way it is supplied by manufacturers (1,000mcg/1ml).

Cyanocobalamin is contraindicated in Leber's disease, may use injectable hydroxocobalamin or methylcobalamin.

Methylcobalamin is thought to be superior in treating neurologic disease.

Only methylcobalamin and hydroxocobalamin should be used in treating inborn errors of B$_{12}$ metabolism.*

Hydroxocobalamin injection 1,000mcg/ml is manufactured by Watson Laboratories, Inc. (Corona, California, phone: 951-493-5300) and is sold by prescription only. NDC 0591-2888-30 (30ml steril multiple dose vial).

Appendix L: Countries in Which Cbl Deficiency Has Been Described in Medical Journals

Belgium	Guatemala	Netherlands	Switzerland
Brazil	Hong Kong	New Zealand	Taiwan
Canada	India	Norway	Thailand
China	Indonesia	Poland	Turkey
Cuba	Israel	Portugal	United Kingdom
Denmark	Italy	Saudi Arabia	United States
Finland	Japan	South Africa	
France	Korea	Spain	
Germany	Kuwait	Sweden	

*Presently there is little literature in medical journals regarding methylcobalamin treatment

Appendix M: Cobalamin Deficiency Criteria List (CDCL)

I. Neurological Manifestations
(+2) paresthesia
(+2) weakness (extremity)
(+2) dizziness, lightheadedness
(+2) syncope
(+2) falling
(+2) abnormal gait/ataxia
(+2) mental status change
(+2) confusion/disorientation
(+2) dementia
(+2) diminished proprioception
(+2) distorted touch/pain perception
(+2) impaired vibration sense
(+2) muscular spasticity
(+2) tremor
(+2) +Babinski or +Lhermitte's sign
(+2) paralysis
(+1) incontinence (urinary/fecal)
(+1) impotence

II. Hematologic Manifestations Deficiency
(+2) anemia
(+2) macrocytosis
(+2) ovalocytes or eliptocytes
(+2) neutrophil hypersegmentation
(+1) anisocytosis
(+1) leukopenia
(+1) thrombocytopenia
(+1) microcytosis

III. Psychiatric Manifestations
(+2) depression
(+2) hallucinations
(+2) delusions
(+2) violent behavior
(+2) personality changes
(+2) psychosis
(+2) apathy
(+2) paranoia
(+2) irritability
(+2) schizophrenia

IV. Gastrointestinal Diseases
(+2) gastric atrophy
(+2) hypochlorhydria/achlorhydria
(+2) gastritis
(+2) ulcers
(+2) inflammatory bowel disease
(+2) diverticulosis
(+2) gastrointestinal neoplasms
(+2) gastrointestinal resections
(+2) malabsorption syndromes
(+2) small bowel overgrowth
(+2) diphyllobothrium infection
(+2) Zollinger-Ellison syndrome
(+2) pancreatic exocrine insufficiency
(+2) Imerslund-Gräesbeck syndrome
(+2) Crohn's disease (regional enteritis)
(+2) Celiac disease (gluten enteropathy)

(+2) GERD

V. Population at Risk
(+1) age sixty years or greater
(+2) family history of pernicious anemia
(+2) Eating disorders (anorexia, bulemia)
(+2) gastric bypass
(+1) history of thyroid disorders
(+1) history of autoimmune disorders
(+1) history of IDDM
(+1) history of cancer, chemotherapy, or
    radiation therapy
(+1) administration of nitrous oxide
(+2) vegans or vegetarians
(+1) prescribed medications: (antacids, H2-blockers,
    potassium chloride, phenytoin, metformin, proton
    pump inhibitors, cholestyramine, colchicine)
(+1) on folic acid therapy

VI. Disorders with Possible Underlying Cbl Deficiency*
(+2) Alzheimer's disease
(+2) multiple sclerosis
(+2) peripheral neuropathies
(+2) AIDS dementia complex
(+2) hyperhomocysteinemia
(+2) congestive heart failure
(+2) autism
(+2) fibromyalgia
(+2) patients on hemodialysis
(+2) vertigo
(+2) Meniere's disease
(+2) infertility
(+2) chronic fatigue syndrome
(+1) history of occlusive vascular disorders
    (TIA, CVA, MI, PE, DVT)
(+1) thalassemia trait
(+1) iron deficiency
(+1) alcoholism
(+1) polycythemia
(+1) radiculopathy from back disorder/injury
(+1) chronic pain with drug seeking behavior

VII. Other Manifestations of Cbl Deficiency
(+1) fatigue/lack of energy
(+1) generalized weakness
(+1) weight loss/loss of appetite
(+1) constipation or diarrhea
(+1) optic neuritis
(+1) orthostatic hypotension
(+1) chest pain/exertional dyspnea
(+1) hepatomegaly or splenomegaly
(+1) poor wound healing/ulcer/decubitus
(+1) premature graying
(+1) hyperpigmentation
(+1) pallor
(+1) glossitis
(+1) tinnitus
(+1) vitiligo
(+1) cervical dysplasia

*(Some of these disorders/conditions can be mistakenly
diagnosed in cases where symptoms actually stem from B12
deficiency. Others, such as hemodialysis, can contribute to the
risk of B12 deficiency. In a number of these conditions, B12
deficiency needs to be investigated as an underlying cause.)

Cobalamin Deficiency Risk (CDR) Score
Low risk: less than 3. Moderate risk: 3 to 6.
High risk: more than 6

Appendix N: Laboratory Data of 12 Patients Presenting to a Community ED with Symptoms of Vitamin B_{12} Deficiency

norms		211-911 pg/ml	4.5-11 x1000/ mm3	11.7-15.7 gm/dl	34.9-46.9%	80.5-99.7fL	11.5-14.5%		
case #	age/sex	B_{12}	WBC	HgB	HCT	MCV	RDW	chief complaint	CDR score
1.*	44 F	185	8.4	10.7	31.8	80.7	15.6	syncope/trauma	12
2.*	51 F	211	6.5	6.8	20.3	97.9	16.2	dyspnea/weakness	11
3.	77 F	168	7.9	12.9	37.9	88.0	14.2	chest pain	10
4.	82 F	210	20.2	10.9	32.9	88.6	17.6	weakness (r. side)	11
5.	89 F	156	4.4	12.2	35.5	102.5	12.3	fall - Fx wrist	9
6.*	52 F	146	4.6	11.4	33.5	109.8	15.5	abd. & back pain	18
7.	69 F	165	11.3	10.1	15.2	65.8	15.2	chest pain	11
8.	77 F	170	7.4	10.4	32.2	85.0	18.0	chest pain	16
9.*	57 F	186	3.1	14.3	41.1	92.1	12.8	left arm tremor	8
10.	59 F	172	3.9	12.9	40.6	87.6	14.4	fatigue/weakness	11
11.	51 F		2.9	6.3	19.0	136.3	32.2	severe fatigue	12
12.	19 F	240	7.52	14.6	43.9	102.2	15.4	elevated MCV	5

Blank boxes: data not available
(*): Patient has history of thyroid disorder.
The first eight patients were from a 50-patient study from the Hospital A emergency department, each had a Cobalamin Deficiency Risk (CDR) Score of three or more. Patients 9, 10, and 11 were not tallied in the percentages of the 50-patient study, for they presented after the 50-patient sample was collected. Patient 11 had a family history of pernicious anemia, and was treated with B_{12} injections intermittently by her family doctor. Her MMA was 1.19 mcmol/L (normal less than 0.4), Hcy 17 mcmol/L (normal less than 15). Patient 12 presented before the 50-patient sample was started. Patient 12 was worked up and diagnosed with autoimmune pernicious anemia by a hematologist.

Results:
1. 8/50 (16%) were found to have subnormal serum vitamin B12 levels.
2. 10/50 (20%) were found to have serum B_{12} levels from 212 to 350pg/ml.
3. 18/50 (36%) were found to have serum B_{12} levels below 350pg/ml which warranted further workup.

Deficient patients in fifty patient study:
8/8 (100%) were female   3/8 (38%) had thyroid disorders
5/8 (62.5%) were anemic   6/8 (75%) had decreased HCT
2/8 (25%) were macrocytic   1/8 (12.5%) was microcytic
5/8 (62.5%) had elevated RDW   1/8 (12.5%) was anemic and macrocytic
5/8 (62.5%) were over age sixty

Appendix O: Laboratory Data from Hospital Z (Serum Vitamin B12 <180pg/ml); Forty Patients Presenting to a Community ED Using CDCL and CDR Score

	norms	180-914 pg/ml	M: 4.3-5.5 F: 3.7-5.3 mm3	M: 12.3-16.9 F: 11.4-15.9 gm/dl	M: 40-50 F: 34.8-46 %	80-100 fl	11.9-15.1 %		
case #	age/sex	B12	RBC	HGB	HCT	MCV	RDW	chief complaint	CDR Score
1.*	42 F	134	4.46	13.3	38.3	85.9	12.1	chest pain	4
2.	46 F	177	4.83	13.7	41.8	86.5	17.1	chest pain	10
3.	54 F	131	1.37	5.5	15.2	111.2	21.1	unresponsive/fall	19
4.	59 M	157	5.94	16.0	48.0	80.9	14.4	seizure	5
5.	61 M	136	4.71	15.6	46.4	98.5	15.3	chest pain	6
6.	62 F	164	4.67	13.7	40.5	86.6	13.5	chronic back pain with radiculopathy	15
7.	69 M	143	4.59	15.7	45.7	99.5	11.8	dizziness/headache	10
8.*	74 F	107	5.05	14.9	44.5	88.0	14.5	syncope, (?) seizure	13
9.	74 F	151	3.99	10.7	32.5	81.4	13.8	chest pain	5
10.	78 M	167	3.44	10.4	31.6	91.7	13.6	weakness/TIA	7
11.*	79 F	90	3.19	11.7	34.7	108.5	19.0	dizziness/fall	10
12.*	80 M	84	4.33	14.2	41.9	96.5	13.6	right arm weakness with numbness	10
13.*	80 M	137	4.13	12.7	36.7	88.9	12.9	syncope	8
14.	81 F	99	4.46	11.5	34.4	77.0	16.5	TIA/fall/weakness	10
15.	81 F	161	4.44	14.2	42.3	95.0	13.9	weakness	14
16.*	82 F	147	2.82	8.6	25.2	89.2	14.0	light headedness	13
17.	82 F	93	3.39	10.3	30.1	88.6	13.0	dizziness, fall	13
18.	83 F	166	3.91	12.2	36.2	92.4	14.3	cellulitis lower extremity	7
19.	86 M	131	4.26	12.9	37.4	87.7	13.6	fall	6
20.*	86 M	89	3.95	11.6	34.3	86.8	13.5	weakness/fall	12
21.	87M	159	2.31	7.5	22.4	97.0	14.0	fall, left hip Fx	16
22.*	87 F	180	3.48	10.8	31.4	90.0	13.5	dyspnea, weakness	14
23.	89 F	179	4.50	13.4	40.5	90.1	13.1	unresponsive	8
24.*	92 F	132	3.59	11.3	32.8	91.2	12.1	fall, rib Fx	11

Laboratory Data from Hospital Z
(Serum Vitamin B$_{12}$ 181~211pg/ml)

case #	age/sex	B$_{12}$	RBC	HGB	HCT	MCV	RDW	chief complaint	CDR Score
25.	35 F	192	4.34	9.7	30.3	69.8	15.5	chest pain	5
26.	39 M	208	4.22	14.8	43.0	101.8	12.1	headache	3
27.	44 F	200	3.35	11.5	33.6	100.1	12.6	abdominal pain	2
28.	52 M	194	4.45	15.3	44.6	100.1	12.3	chest pain	11
*29.	66 F	208	3.74	10.3	30.8	82.1	12.4	DVT/cellulitis	10
30.	66 M	208	4.83	15.6	46.1	95.3	13.1	abdominal pain, constipation	5
31.	69 F	205	3.62	10.3	31.4	86.7	15.2	fall/right hip fracture	15
*32.	70 F	194	4.73	13.9	40.7	85.9	14.1	mental status change	16
33.	73 M	210	4.67	15.0	43.7	93.6	13.1	syncopal episode	9
34.	74 F	198	4.36	13.5	39.3	90.2	11.8	abdominal pain	7
35.	77 F	190	4.26	13.2	39.0	91.4	13.4	dizziness, fall x 2	13
36.	79 F	199	4.13	11.8	35.2	85.2	14.2	cellulitis right foot	7
37.	82 F	203	4.80	14.8	43.9	91.6	13.6	syncope, confusion, gait disorder	11
38.	82 M	207	4.47	9.1	28.8	64.3	18.6	dyspnea, new onset of atrial fibrillation	7
39.	88 M	187	4.47	14.2	42.4	94.8	13.7	weakness, fell six months ago - Fx L5	12
40.	90 F	205	4.01	12.8	38.2	95.4	13.3	right sided weakness	9

25/40 (62.5%) female
15/40 (37.5%) male
5/40 (12.5%) macrocytic
1/40 (.03%) macrocytic anemia
3/40 (.05%) microcytic
1/40 (.03%) microcytic anemia
13/40 (32.5%) anemic
24/40 (60%) decreased hematocrit
10/40 (25%) elevated RDW

8/40 (21%) were < 60 years   6/40 (15%) chest pain
10/40 (25%) CHF
10/40 (25%) thyroid disease (designated with *symbol)
8/40 (21%) dementia
9/40 (23%) psychiatric disorder
24/40 (60%) neurologic manifestation
18/40 (45%) TIA/CVA
15/40 (38%) fell or fell within the past year
15/40 (38%) H2-blocker/anti-secretory proton pump inhibitor

Appendix P: Reasons Physicians Do Not Screen for or Treat Vitamin B$_{12}$ Deficiency

Knowledge deficit (believing it's only a hematologic disorder)
Not up-to-date with current literature; past prejudices
Fear of patients incurring cost of tests; fear of not being reimbursed
Do not believe it is their specialty's job or responsibility to screen for it
Resistance to change
Do not believe it is cost effective or needed
Not familiar with reimbursement codes
Believe too much effort in following up with patient's results (contacting family
    physician or patient)
Ego
Apathy, laziness
Overworked, disinterested in adding another disease process to rule out
Fear of forgetting to follow up with patient results and therefore increased liability

Appendix Q: Substandard Care

Telling patients they do not require parenteral B12 therapy when they have been receiving
    injections for years
Obtaining a serum B$_{12}$ level to disprove a patient's need, months or years after the patient
    has started receiving injections
Assuming a patient cannot have B$_{12}$ deficiency because he or she is not anemic or macrocytic
Not working up a patient for B$_{12}$ deficiency when anemia or macrocytosis is present
Not inquiring about a patient's B$_{12}$ status when neurologic or psychiatric manifestations are
    present
Prescribing medications before ruling out B$_{12}$ deficiency
Not screening elderly and at-risk patients in general
Not screening elderly and at-risk patients pre-operatively
Making the diagnosis of dementia without ruling out B$_{12}$ deficiency
Institutionalizing an elder in a nursing home before ruling out B$_{12}$ deficiency
Assuming an elder's signs and symptoms are caused by preexisting diseases, therefore not
    contemplating B$_{12}$ deficiency
Diagnosing B$_{12}$ deficiency late when severe anemia has developed, requiring blood
    transfusions
Improper treatment
    not giving monthly injections of B$_{12}$ for life
    inconsistently giving B$_{12}$ injections
    not giving the series of injections to rebuild a patient's store, when the patient is
        determined to have pernicious anemia or B$_{12}$ deficiency
    giving patients standard RDA dose of oral B$_{12}$ supplements instead of high-dose (1,000
        mcg) oral therapy or intramuscular injections
    placing patients on chronic antacids, H2-blockers, or anti-secretory proton pump
        inhibitors, and not periodically screening patients for B$_{12}$ deficiency
    not screening for B$_{12}$ deficiency in patients with gastrointestinal diseases (e.g. Crohn's
        disease)
    not treating patients who have undergone gastrointestinal surgeries which induce B$_{12}$
        deficiency
    not ruling out B$_{12}$ deficiency in elderly patients who fall

Appendix R: Diagnostic ICD-9 Reimbursement Codes for Vitamin B$_{12}$ Deficiency

Anemia
281.0 pernicious anemia
281.1 vitamin B$_{12}$ deficiency anemia
281.9 megaloblastic anemia
285.9 unspecified anemia

Neuropathy
355.9 neuropathy (unspecified site)
356.9 peripheral neuropathy
331.7 cerebral degeneration
336.2 subacute combined degeneration of
     spinal cord
781.9 neurological deficit

Other Symptoms
780.7 weakness/lethargy
781.2 gait disturbance
781.3 ataxia and lack of coordination
780.4 dizziness (vertigo)
780.2 syncope
783.2 weight loss

Malabsorption Etiologies
555.2 ileocolitis
555.9 enterocolitis (unspecified site)
579.3 gastrointestinal surgery
579.9 malabsorption not otherwise specified

Dementia
290.0 senile dementia, uncomplicated
290.1 presenile dementia
290.2 senile dementia with depression
294.1 dementia
297.1 paranoid psychosis, chronic
297.9 paranoid state, unspecified
300.9 mental status change
331.0 Alzheimer's disease/dementia

Deficiency
266.2 vitamin B$_{12}$ or folate deficiency
266.9 unspecified vitamin B-complex deficiency

Most of the above categories were taken from Norman Clinical Laboratory, Inc. test request form, uses ICD-9 codes.

Appendix S: Cost (2005) of Tests to Diagnose Vitamin B12 Deficiency

CBC	$35.00
Serum B$_{12}$	$60.00
Serum MMA	$189.70
Urine MMA	$70.00 Norman Clinical Lab
	$203.40 Mayo Clinic Labs
	Other labs also offer this service at various prices
Serum Hcy	$111.00
PC Antibody	$86.80
IF Antibody	$101.20
Gastrin	$72.00
Creatinine	$28.00

Sample Case History: In 1999, a fifty-seven-year-old female was diagnosed by a neurologist as having "essential tremor." Blood work ordered by her family doctor (CBC) was sent to her neurologist. A work up for B$_{12}$ deficiency was not done. However, the following tests were performed:

MRI brain w/o contrast:	$1,583.00	
MRI cervical spine w/o contrast	1,583.00	
MSEP + 3 neurology visits:	1,075.00+	(Costs are 1999 U.S. dollars)
Total cost:	$4,241.00	
Patient's cost (20% co-pay):	848.20 -	
Insurance policy paid:	$3,392.80	

This patient also had a history or Hashimoto's thyroiditis. Her son, who is a physician, was urged by us to rule out underlying B$_{12}$ deficiency. Lab results proved autoimmune pernicious anemia. Serum B$_{12}$ was low, MMA and Hcy were elevated, she had a positive parietal cell antibody, and her serum gastrin level was very elevated. After three months of hydroxocobalamin injection therapy, her tremor was 50 percent improved, and her severe left arm weakness was completely resolved. Four years later this patient still has a mild left arm tremor (75 percent reduction). This patient also had abnormal Pap smears for eight years, prior to B$_{12}$ therapy. She had undergone numerous procedures (D&C, LEEP, and bi-annual Pap smears) and was encouraged to have a hysterectomy. Each year since B$_{12}$ therapy was initiated, she has had normal Pap smears.

The cost of the five tests (serum B$_{12}$, serum MMA, gastrin, parietal cell antibody, and creatinine) that resulted in the correct diagnosis of autoimmune pernicious anemia (B$_{12}$ deficiency) was $325.08. Because the patient had a $5.00 co-pay, the cost to her was only $25.00.

Since the test results revealed pernicious anemia, further tests were performed (CBC, Hcy, IF antibody, folate, repeat B$_{12}$). Cost to patient again was $25.00.

Appendix T: Medication Costs (2004)

The following are the costs of drugs patients may be placed on because of psychiatric behavior or other complaints, possibly due to undiagnosed vitamin B12 deficiency:

Drug	Quantity	Cost/ Month	Cost/ Year
Prozac 20mg (1) BID	60	$264.44	$3,173.28
Buspar 5mg (1) TID	90	$96.05	$1,152.60
Serzone 200mg (1) BID	60	$126.31	$1,515.72
Paxil 20mg (1) daily	30	$105.54	$1,266.48
Aricept 5mg (1) daily	30	$170.20	$2,042.40
Antivert 25mg (1) BID	60	$58.33	$699.96
Detrol 1mg (1) daily	30	$68.48	$821.76
Prevacid 30mg (1) daily	30	$135.99	$1,631.88
Prilosec 20mg (1) daily	30	$118.99	$1,427.88
Cyanocobalamin 1,000mcg/month	10ml	$1.00	$12.00
Hydroxocobalamin 1,000mcg/month	30ml	$1.50	$18.00

If a patient was thought to have multiple sclerosis and B_{12} deficiency, or an inborn error of B_{12} metabolism was not ruled out, patients could easily be placed on:

Avonex 30mcg IM once weekly	$1,317.00/month = $15,804.00/year
Betaseron 0.25mg SQ every other day	$1,507.00/month = $18,084.00/year
Copaxone 20mg SQ daily	$1,355.00/month = $16,260.00/year

Appendix U: The Real Cost of Hip Fractures (2003)

Ambulance from home to hospital after a fall	$ 442.00
In-patient hospitalization	
Emergency room services and supplies	1,694.00
Medical supplies	657.00
Surgical supplies and fluoroscopy guidance	1,592.00
Laboratory services	2,920.00
Pharmacy	4,583.00
Respiratory/pulmonary therapy	213.00
X ray/radiology	687.00
Special diagnostics services & supplies	237.00
Orthopedic surgeon fee (ORIF)	2,400.00
(Open reduction internal fixation of femur)	
Anesthesiologist fee	1,024.00
Pre-op holding	793.00
Operating room fee (first thirty minutes)	2,109.00
Operating room fee (remaining OR time)	4,248.00
Recovery room	1,333.00
Room charges (two days)	4,245.00
Occupational and physical therapy evaluations	460.00
	$29,637.00
Post-hospital: rehabilitation	
Room charges (inpatient rehab x fourteen days)	12,390.00
Inpatient rehab services and supplies	7,160.00
Rehabilitation physician fee (for fourteen days)	1,635.00
Home physical therapy sessions (30–60 minutes) nineteen visits	2,185.00
Wheelchair	1,300.00
Bedside commode	120.00
Shower chair (Medicare does not pay)	45.00
Walker	93.00
Four-prong cane	56.00
	$24,984.00

$29,637.00 + $24,984.00 = $54,621.00. Medicare pays 80% of $54,621.00 = $43,696.80. Out of pocket cost for patient, if no other secondary insurance: $10,924.20

Appendix V: Cost of Hospitalization (1999)

(does not include physician and/or surgeon fees—does not include rehabilitation fees)

Diagnosis for Admission	Length of Stay	Cost
1) CHF, hypokalemia, chronic ischemic disease	one day	$3,089.00
2) Right femoral neck fracture (surgically repaired)	three days	$14,487.00
3) Syncope and collapse; distal radius fracture	six days	$16,528.00

Of the $16,528.00 that Medicare approved for the admission of #3, $843.00 was spent for cat scan of the brain without contrast, $1,907.00 for X rays, $1,473.00 for lab, and $210.00 for physical therapy (one evaluation and one visit). This patient was severely vitamin B_{12} deficient and was diagnosed at a cost of $20.00. Could this fall, fracture, and admission have been prevented if this elder had been screened earlier and treated? Physicians, insurance companies, Medicare, and society are willing to pay all of these costs, but are unwilling to screen for B_{12} deficiency to prevent injury, institutionalization, and poor outcomes.

Appendix W: Cost of Institutionalization (1999)

Average assisted living care on memory-impaired unit: $47,400.00/year = $94,800.00/ two years, $237,000.00/five years (not including medications, treatments, or physician fees)

Average base rate for nursing homes: $4,000.00/month = $48,000.00/year = $240,000.00/five years

Additional Costs:

medication administration:	$5.00/day x 365 days =	$1,825.00/year
cognitive impairment:	$15.00/day x 365 days =	$5,475.00/year
mobility management:	$5.00/day x 365 days =	$1,825.00/ year
incontinence:	$12.00/day x 365 days =	$4,380.00/year
dressing assistance:	$6.00/day x 365 days =	$2,190.00/year
		$15,695.00/year
		$48,000.00/year + (base rate)
		$63,695.00/year

Patients' and families' costs average approximately $63,695.00 per year. This comes to $127,390.00 for two years, and $318,475.00 for five years. If five patients went undiagnosed with B_{12} deficiency during one year at one institution, and as a result, were institutionalized, it would cost Medicare, private insurance, patients, their families, and society about $318,475.00 for one year, and $1,592,375.00 to house and care for these five patients for five years. Five patients were found to be B_{12} deficient within a six-week period at the hospital in Appendix N. This study was conducted during one shift, three days per week, on an inconsistent basis. Many patients who needed to be tested were not, due to physician resistance and disinterest. Experts calculated in 1996 that approximately 800,000 Americans over the age of sixty-five had undiagnosed B_{12} deficiency. As more members of the Baby Boomer generation reach sixty-five, this number is likely to rise. It is clear that screening for B_{12} deficiency must become a standard of care.

Appendix X: Treatment Cost (2005)

Vitamin B_{12} (cyanocobalamin) 10ml vial costs $10.00. 1ml/month is needed. $1.00/ month = $12.00 per year, Rx only.

Hydroxocobalamin 30ml vial: Average wholesale price approximately $38. Available from Watson Pharmaceuticals, NDC 0591-2888-30 (1-800-272-5525).

Syringes with needles: Approximately $.25 each. Twelve a year would cost about $3.00

Index

About the Authors

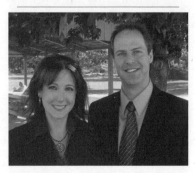

Sally Pacholok, R.N., BSN, an emergency room nurse with eighteen years of experience, received her bachelor's degree in nursing from Wayne State University. Prior to entering the field of nursing, she received an Associate's Degree of Applied Science with magna cum laude honors. She is also an Advanced Emergency Medical Technician (A-EMT), and worked as a paramedic prior to and during nursing school. She has worked in health care for a total of twenty-five years, and has cared for thousands of patients. In addition, she is an Advanced Cardiac Life Support (ACLS) provider, and has assisted instructors at a local community college in training paramedics in ACLS. She is a Trauma Nursing Core Course (TNCC) Provider, an Emergency Nurse Pediatric Course (ENPC) Provider, and a member of the Emergency Nurses Association (ENA).

In 1985, Pacholok diagnosed herself with vitamin B_{12} deficiency, after her doctors had failed to identify her condition. As a result, she is passionate about the need to educate the public about the dangerous consequences of this hidden and all-too-common disease.

Jeffrey J. Stuart, D.O., a physician who has practiced emergency medicine for twelve years, is board certified in this field. He is also certified in Advanced Trauma Life Support, Advanced Cardiac Life Support (ACLS), Advanced Pediatric Life Support, and Neonatal Resuscitation. Stuart received his Doctor of Osteopathy degree from the Chicago College of Osteopathic Medicine. His training includes field amputation and hazardous materials decontamination, and he has also participated in training sessions with the Detroit Metropolitan Airport SWAT team. Dr. Stuart participated in visual brain research at the National Institute of Mental Health in Bethesda, Maryland, in 1987, and was involved in cholesterol metabolism research at the Rockefeller University Hospital in New York City in 1985. He is a member of the American Osteopathic Association, the American College of Osteopathic Emergency Physicians, the Macomb County Osteopathic Society, and the Michigan Osteopathic Association.